Foreword

I was pleased to be able to support the preparation of this handbook with Regional R&D funding. One of our priorities in the NW is to extend the range of professionals and health care settings involved in health related research. To build capacity and to give people confidence to participate in research, we need to provide researchers with a variety of support tools and this handbook is an excellent starting point for new and aspiring researchers. The regional R&D office provides other support and training through bursaries, fellowships, support units and project funding schemes which are referenced in the handbook. This handbook doesn't attempt to replace the many excellent texts which deal in depth with the technical and scientific aspects of health services research which researchers may still need to consult. It aims to be a helpful starting point.

The handbook describes the NHS R&D strategy and its context so that researchers can begin to develop their ideas and provides pointers and pathways for researchers to follow. It places an appropriate emphasis on the ethical and design aspects of research and encourages researchers to think from the outset about how they will communicate and use the results of their research: a crucial aspect which sadly is often neglected even by the most eminent of researchers.

Whilst the language of the handbook tries to avoid jargon, there is an excellent glossary of the terms commonly used by health service researchers in the notes. I would encourage researchers to read this handbook, whether they need general guidance or help on a particular aspect of their research.

Finally, I would like to thank the editorial team for their time and interest in producing this handbook for the benefit of the NHS in the NW.

Professor Maggie Pearson

North West Regional Director of Research and Development

Acknowledgements

This book has been produced with the help of funding from the Research and Development (R&D) Directorate of the NHS Executive North West. The development of the book was overseen by an editorial board whose contribution throughout the many stages and revisions is gratefully acknowledged. A list of the board members is included at the end of the handbook. The book also includes contributions from a number of sources and individuals, which are referenced appropriately in the text. In particular, the work by Selvi Jeyaseelan, John Bevans and Tracy Watson was invaluable to ensure that the book was written and compiled to meet the objectives defined by the editorial board. The help of many individuals in reviewing the various drafts and in the final evaluation is also acknowledged.

Keith T Chantler

Editor

CONTENTS

FOREWORD i

ACKNOWLEDGEMENTS ii

INTRODUCTION 3

How to Use this Guide 4
Updating the Guide 5

1) THE ORGANISATION AND FUNDING OF RESEARCH IN THE NHS 7

National R&D Strategy 7
Need for consumer involvement in R&D 8
Need for Multidisciplinary Work 9
How Research is Organised in the NHS Regions 10
References 11

2) THE ROLE OF THE HEALTH PROFESSIONAL 13

Research Priorities in the NHS 14
Project Resources 14
Reference 15

3) DEVELOPING YOUR RESEARCH IDEA 17

Undertaking a Review of the Existing Literature 18
Local Access Computer Search of CD-ROM Databases 19
Manual Searching through Journals 20
Internet 21
Choosing an Appropriate Research Methodology 25
Statistics and Health Economics 28
References 30

4) WRITING A RESEARCH PROPOSAL 33

Protocol Contents 34
Development Protocol 38
References 38

5) ETHICAL CONSIDERATIONS 41

Overview 42
Role of the Local Research Ethics Committee 42
Application Procedure 42
Points to Consider 44
Multi-Centre Trials 45
Research on Animals 45
References 45

6) CLINICAL INDEMNITY AND LEGAL ISSUES 47

Clinical Risks 48
Contracts for Research 48
References 49

7) FUNDING THE COSTS OF YOUR RESEARCH 51

Submitting Grant Applications 52
Responsibilities for Research Funds 53
Sources of Funding 54
The National Health Service Funding Schemes 54
Other National Funding Sources 54
References 56

8) PROJECT MANAGEMENT AND PERFORMANCE 57

Time Management 58
Staffing of Research Projects 61
Budget Management 62
Reviewing the Project 65

9) PRESENTING YOUR RESEARCH FINDINGS 67

Methods of Dissemination 69
References 70

10) USING RESEARCH EVIDENCE 73

Development and the Development Protocol 74
Critical Evaluation and Appraisal of Research 75
References 76

APPENDIX A: PRINCIPLES GOVERNING THE ALLOCATION OF FUNDS FROM THE NHS R&D LEVY 79

APPENDIX B: OTHER FUNDING SOURCES 83

Postal Addresses and Telephone Numbers 83
Web Site Addresses 83

APPENDIX C: THE NATIONAL R&D PRIORITY AREAS 85

GLOSSARY OF TERMS USED IN RESEARCH 87

BIBLIOGRAPHY 93

EDITORIAL BOARD 99

INTRODUCTION

The National Health Service (NHS) is funded from public money. All those who work in the NHS have a duty to use these funds efficiently and effectively. Like many public and private organisations, all sectors of the NHS are expected to deliver high quality services, whilst the available resources are subject to competing priorities. Due to increasing pressure on these resources, there is a need to:

- Improve service provision
- Improve all aspects of clinical and organisational efficiency
- Enhance clinical and managerial decision-making
- Ensure the effective use of NHS resources.

In the NHS, our business is treating and caring for patients. It is vitally important that, when we make decisions to change the way in which we deliver care, we do so on the basis of facts. To do this we need a process in which proposed changes, improvements and new ideas can be tested (research), evaluated and put into service (development). The NHS recognises that it needs to invest in research to ensure that the care that its doctors, dentists and nurses deliver is the most up-to-date and effective.

The NHS currently invests around £450 million p.a. to fund the direct costs of research, e.g. laboratory tests, surveys and purchase of equipment. It also funds the indirect costs, sometimes called the infrastructure costs, such as the buildings and the time of staff to carry out research. The research funding that the NHS provides is subject to the same cost pressures as other NHS resources and it is the responsibility of every researcher to be able to demonstrate that the outcomes of research provide a good return on the public money invested.

Many people working in the NHS have ideas how to make improvements in the work they do and would like to initiate some research, but feel they lack the necessary skills, or are unsure of how to begin. In Universities, Trusts and libraries, there are volumes of literature describing different research methodologies, statistics and research ethics. Sometimes, however, the literature is too specific and in many cases fails to address the answer to the range of questions which the new researcher needs answers to.

This guide has been specifically designed to provide an introduction to the context in which health services research is carried out and the fundamentals of the research process. It aims to give new and aspiring researchers confidence to embark upon their own research and development and acts as a reference point for more experienced researchers.

How to Use this Guide

The book comprises a series of chapters which broadly correspond with the life cycle of a typical research project. However, each chapter is designed to stand alone and to provide the reader with an introduction to a particular aspect of the research process. Each chapter has:

- A list of **key** points
- A **checklist** which you might use to review your own project or idea
- A **bibliography** of useful references.

The guide aims to provide the researcher with advice and guidance in the following areas:

- Definitions of research, development and implementation
- National, regional and local NHS R&D structures
- Sources of advice and support which are available to facilitate quality research
- Basics of the research process.

The following important topics are discussed in more depth:

- Ethics and the Ethics Committee approval processes
- Implementing the results of research.

The book aims to provide an understanding of the research process, gives guidance on statistical awareness and includes a comprehensive glossary of terminology to enable the reader to start undertaking research. It introduces evaluation and critical appraisal of research findings, which are important techniques used to implement the results of your own or others' research. These are skills which can be learned by practice and participation. An effective way to do this is through collaborating with other more experienced researchers and by regular interaction with others who are interested in the same topics.

Updating the Guide

It is not feasible to keep a printed book up-to-date. However, using the Internet, it is possible to do this electronically. You can access the latest version of this guide on the NHSnet. This contains new references and current funding information.

NOTE: Research and development are recognised as separate activities, but are generally organised and funded in the same ways in the NHS. They are referred to as 'research' in the text except where there is an intention or need to differentiate them. Implementation of research is not funded in the same way; this is the responsibility of Trusts and Health Authorities through clinical care budgets. We have used the term 'Trust' to denote all types of NHS Trust, both acute and community, and, where applicable, other NHS settings such as primary care.

1 THE ORGANISATION AND FUNDING OF RESEARCH IN THE NHS

- National R&D strategy
- Regional organisation of research
- Local organisation of research

National R&D Strategy

Historically, research activity in the NHS was largely confined to medical research in large teaching hospitals often associated with a University Medical or Dental School. Changes in clinical practice due to technological development and the re-organisation of the NHS (resulting from the NHS and Community Care Act 1990) have increased the focus of health care delivered in the community. These two important driving forces have created a need to change the location and nature of research in the NHS. The publication of the NHS R&D Strategy in 1991 set out for the first time a national R&D strategy. Details of the R&D Strategy can be found at the Department of Health Web site: (http://www.open.gov.uk/doh/rdd1.htm).

The aim of the NHS R&D Strategy is to '*improve the health of the nation by promoting a knowledge-based health service in which clinical, managerial and policy decisions are informed by sound information about research findings and scientific developments. It is concerned with both the development of new practice and understanding existing practice. It is essential that research findings are accessible and implemented through the integration of research with other NHS activities.*'

The various components of the research and development process can be defined as follows;

- **Research** - scientific activity to test hypotheses and thus generate knowledge which may subsequently be useful in improving the effectiveness or efficiency of health care
- **Development** - experimental introduction into practice of alternative clinical procedures or methods of care, together with the simultaneous evaluation of their effectiveness or efficiency or both
- **Dissemination** - making available research-based information to

practitioners and decision-makers within the NHS in order to enhance opportunities for changing behaviour

- **Implementation** - establishment in routine practice of (clinical) procedures or methods (of care) for which there is evidence of effectiveness and efficiency. Implementation work will be in areas where the results of research or development are available but work needs to be conducted on the practical steps necessary to ensure that the benefits of the research or development are secured in general.

The NHS Director of R&D commissioned a review of the organisation and funding of R&D in England. The Report of the NHS R&D Task Force (Culyer Report), produced in 1994, set out five broad principles for supporting research in the NHS:

- Single national funding source for research (**R&D Levy**)
- **No cross-subsidies** between patient care and research
- Service Increment for Teaching and Research (SIFTR) allocation replaced by **competitive bids** for funding
- Emphasis on **outcomes** and **performance**
- Emphasis on **collaboration** and **partnership**.

The last principle emphasises the need to encourage the involvement of a wider range of health professionals in health services research in a variety of health service settings and also patients as consumers of the outputs of the research.

Need for consumer involvement in R&D

Over the last few years the NHS has been placing increasing importance on the views of users (patients) in developing services and policies; this includes the National R&D Strategy. A Standing Advisory Group on Consumer Involvement in the NHS R&D Programme has been established which produced its first report in January 1998 entitled "Research: What's in it for consumers".

Consumer involvement does not simply refer to the consumers being the "*subject of the research - instead consumer involvement is the active involvement of consumers in the research process...(occurring) in any or all of the processes involved in research - setting the research agenda, commissioning research, undertaking research, interpreting research and disseminating the results".*

The benefits of involving consumers has been politically mandated with the following benefits identified:

- It is believed that by involving consumers the research will be more relevant and reliable as the consumers are users of the service and know the service best.
- Consumers often have knowledge and expertise that complement those of health care professionals and researchers; this may improve the quality of the research.
- Consumers will benefit too in that they will develop an understanding of the need for research and the potential benefits to patient care.

The involvement of the consumer throughout is not easy and is not consistent with how research has been prioritised and conducted in the past:

- Consumers/patients who are involved are rarely typical and input may be biased or partial. It is likely that they will not have any medical knowledge or expertise in scientific methods.
- Consumers interests may be assumed to be adequately represented by the healthcare professional, therefore there is a duplication of effort. This is not always believed to be the case, and it is open to question whether all professionals understand their patients' perspective.

Although consumer involvement is much advocated, it is important that it is put into context. Consumer involvement may vary depending on the type of research, and it should be used where there is a potential added benefit rather than an act of tokenism. It is important that consumer involvement should be evaluated in each case.

Need for Multidisciplinary Work

The NHS recognises that the delivery of health care is not the province of any single profession; it is delivered by many professionals working together in teams. It seems natural then that there should be an emphasis on multidisciplinary teams to carry out research. There should also be wide participation in identifying research needs and priorities. All health care disciplines and service settings should be reflected in the scope of research in the NHS.

Building on the recommendations of the Culyer report, the NHS published the NHS R&D Strategic Framework in January 1997. This sets out the principles under which the NHS will support and fund clinical research. These principles are that all research whose costs are met with NHS funds should:

- Provide the **new knowledge** necessary to improve the performance of the NHS in improving the health of the nation
- Be designed so that the results are **generalisable** (useful to those with a similar problem)
- Follow a **well-written protocol**
- Be based on a **peer-reviewed** protocol
- Have obtained (where necessary) **approval** from the Local Research Ethics Committee and any other relevant bodies
- Have clear arrangements for **project management**
- Plan to **report findings**, usually in the form of a publication. This will allow the findings to be critically appraised and accessible to those who could benefit from them.

These criteria should be fulfilled if direct funding is provided by the NHS; it is also good practice that these criteria are fulfilled for any research.

How Research is Organised in the NHS Regions

The Culyer report recommends that '*the Regional Offices' Director of Research & Development should be the focal point for R&D within each region.*'

Each Regional Office of the NHS is responsible for:

- Providing funding to support proposals that will enable researchers to conduct high quality research which is of value to the NHS, e.g. provision of bursaries and R&D funding
- Providing advice and support to researchers applying for funding
- Advising on possible methods to facilitate the development of research capability and capacity and increase the quality of research
- Identifying R&D priorities so that the NHS can commission research to address problems which are important and relevant to the Service.

In the North West of England, the Regional Office's R&D Directorate aims to develop the R&D capability of professional groups, disciplines and NHS organisations which are presently under-represented. Funding is available for various research topics from fundamental research to the rigorous study of the application of new knowledge in service settings. Provided the research area is relevant to the NHS, there are no areas that are ineligible for funding. However, for commissioned work, those projects which come under one of the agreed national or regional priorities will be given preference, (these are updated regularly, for further details on regional priorities please contact your Regional Office).

Local Organisation of Research

It is likely that your Trust will have a Research Strategy or Plan. This will describe the major research groups in your Trust and their research plans. These plans will take account of the research needs of your Trust to support its service activities and will be based upon the capacity of your Trust, in terms of patients and the infrastructure to support research. You should be aware of these plans and the way in which your Trust organises its research. Many Trusts have either R&D offices or co-ordinators responsible for R&D; they will provide you with help and advice on how to start and pursue your research.

Your local Health Authority and Primary Care Groups will have their own R&D priorities; these are reviewed regularly and are included in their Service and Financial Frameworks and Health Improvement Programmes. Your Trust will discuss with the Health Authority its overall R&D plans and there is no requirement for you to discuss your individual project with the Health Authority. If, however, your project will involve large numbers of patients or will have significant ongoing costs after the research has finished, it may be prudent to alert them to the consequences. Health Authorities do commission research work themselves; it may be that your proposals will fit into one of their priority areas and this will be a potential source of funding. In the North West, you can get information on these areas from the R&D section of your Health Authority.

References

Supporting Research and Development in the NHS: A Report to the Minister for Health by a Research and Development Task Force chaired by Professor Anthony Culyer. HMSO 1994

Strategic Framework for the Use of the NHS R&D Levy. NHS Executive 1997

Research: What's in it for consumers? First report of the Standing Advisory Committee on Consumer Involvement in the NHS R&D Programme, Report to the Central Research and Development Committee 1996/97

Checklist

1. Does the proposed research project:
    - Have a research team with the appropriate skills, resources and facilities to carry out the research?
    - Provide new knowledge relevant to the needs of your Trust or the NHS?
    - Produce generalisable results?
    - Follow a clear protocol?

Will it be:

- Peer-reviewed?
- Approved by the appropriate Ethics Committee?

2. Will it have clear arrangements for project management?
3. How do you plan to report your findings?

2) THE ROLE OF THE HEALTH PROFESSIONAL

- Choosing a research topic
- Research priorities in the NHS
- Project resources

To ensure that the NHS provides the best and most effective services, all groups and individuals are encouraged to review critically how services are provided and to suggest ways in which they can be improved. Research, therefore, is not limited to any single professional group working in the NHS and it is essential that we base the decisions which shape our services on sound research evidence. It follows therefore that the research we carry out in the NHS should be directed at improving services, i.e. it should be relevant to our work.

There are no defined rules or processes which govern the selection or identification of a research question. The questions most often arise from problems encountered during working life, from discussion with colleagues or patients or from reading the results of other published research. The NHS, like any other organisation, recognises the need for research to develop its services; in the case of the NHS, it is not to make a bigger profit, but to provide better, more effective and more appropriate health care services. The funding available to support research is limited and so choices must be made and the NHS has set out the principles which govern all NHS funds used to support research. These principles are fully described in Executive Letter (97)77 and a summary is included in Appendix A.

Each principle is important in its own right, but some will apply more readily to individual projects rather than large programmes. The following points are examples of the principles which will apply to all projects large and small:

- **Multidisciplinary** - Your research should include the most effective mix of individuals and expertise which will ensure that the research is well designed, conducted and reported. This may well include NHS and University staff among others in the public and private sectors.

- **Quality and relevance** - The proposed research should be of good quality and should aim to provide a cost-effective answer to the particular question. There is a broad spectrum of research which is relevant to the

NHS, ranging from laboratory research to health services, or clinical, research, all of which will help to provide evidence upon which best practice can be based.

Research Priorities in the NHS

The NHS Executive Headquarters has responsibility for commissioning R&D nationally and will provide funds to commission high quality research which is relevant to the development of its services. The national programmes can be grouped under three main headings - the Health Technology Assessment (HTA) programme, Service Delivery and Organisation (SDO) programme and the New and Emerging Application of Technology (NEAT) programme. Information on current priorities is included in Appendix C, and the most up-to-date information can be obtained from the R&D Department at the Department of Health[1].

In the eight geographical regions of the NHS, the R&D departments of the Regional Offices consult widely to develop sets of priorities which include research topic areas which may be specific to their populations. A particular priority is to ensure that as many individuals and groups as possible have the confidence, skill, expertise and infrastructure support to participate in research to improve services.

At a local level, Health Authorities, working with their colleagues in public health departments and using information from the various national review centres, incorporate their R&D priorities into their regular discussions with providers. Health Authorities in the North West are required to include their R&D priorities in their annual purchasing plans and strategic and financial framework documents. Your own Trust's R&D manager or the R&D co-ordinator at the Health Authority will advise you of the current list of priorities.

Project Resources

There are many sources of funding for research which do not specify any particular priority area, e.g. the Medical Research Council and Wellcome Trust. Whatever your proposed research area, you must ensure that what you plan to do

---

[1] Website: http://www.open.gov.uk/doh/rddl.htm; Address: R&D, Room 402A, Department of Health, Skipton House, 80 London road, London SE1 6LH; Tel: 0171 972 1659; Fax: 0171 972 1700

fits in with the research plans and priorities of the organisation where the research will be carried out. If not, the resources that you need to undertake your research may not be available to you.

In simple terms, to carry out clinical research, you must be certain that the patients that you need for your research are within the normal referral patterns to your Trust. If not, then it is unlikely that your Trust would provide support without explicit agreement from your Health Authorities unless the study is fully funded by your research sponsor.

As you begin to formulate your research question, consider what happens at the end of your research project. You should plan how you will let others know about the results of your research. The end produce of your research project, Master's degree or PhD should not be just another book on the shelf.

Reference

Executive Letter (97)77: Meeting Patient Costs Associated with R&D in the NHS

Checklist

1. Will your research lead to improved services?
2. Is it multidisciplinary?
3. Does it aim to provide a cost-effective answer to the research question?
4. Does the project fit in with the research plans and priorities of the organisation?
5. Can you identify a source of funding?

3) DEVELOPING YOUR RESEARCH IDEA

- Literature reviews
- Searching CD-ROM databases
- Internet
- Research methodology
- Statistics
- Health economics
- Intellectual property

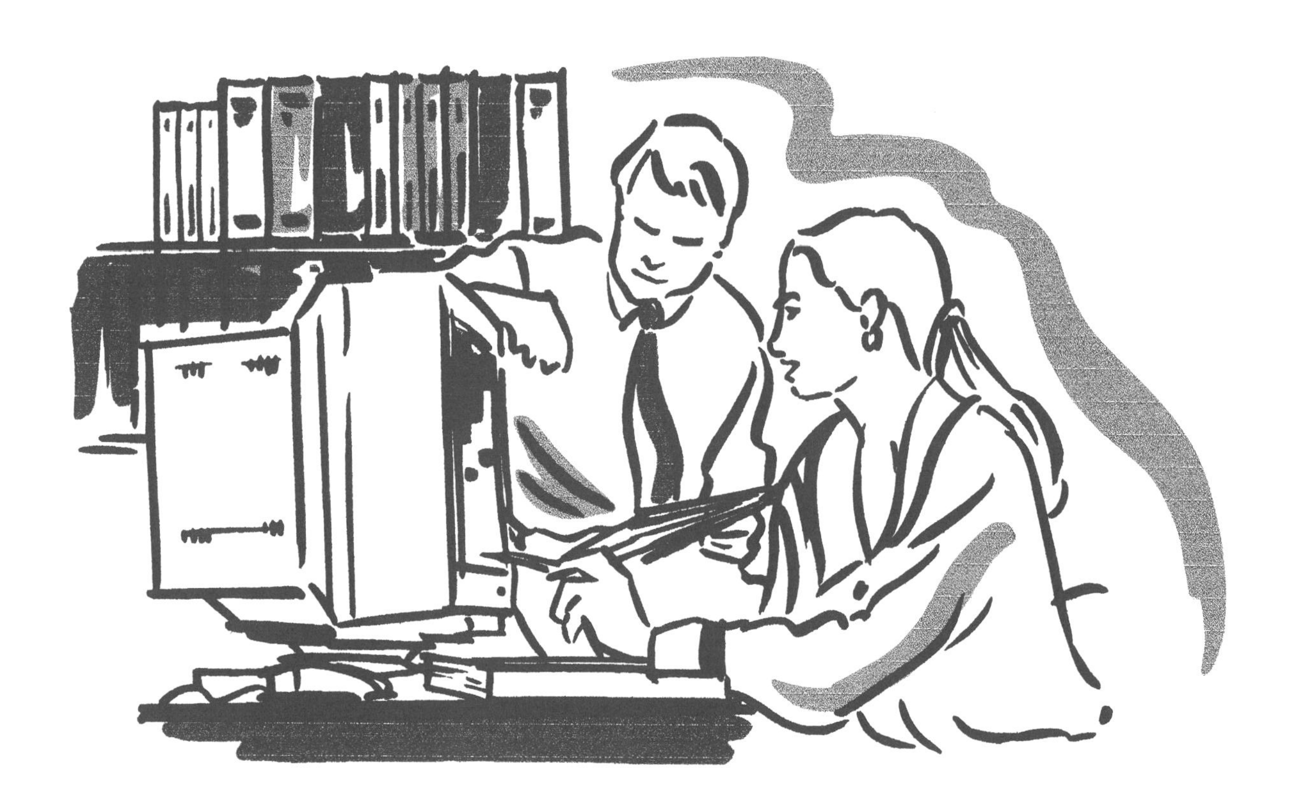

There are a number of important components in the identification, development and refinement of a basic research idea, and its conversion into a feasible research study. The component parts typical of most research projects are:

- Undertaking a review of the existing literature
- Accessing advice
- Choosing an appropriate research methodology
- Seeking specialist advice (statistics and health economics).

Undertaking a Review of the Existing Literature

When you have formulated your research question, often referred to as the hypothesis, a review of all the relevant literature (i.e. professional journal papers, research reports, books, etc.) concerning the area to be investigated should be carried out. The purpose of this task is:

- To improve your understanding of the research area
- To ensure that your proposed study has not already been conducted
- To give you an idea of other methods and techniques that could be employed in your study.

When conducting your review, initially you should aim to cover broad topics associated with your area of research; the searches can then be made more specific as you begin to form a clearer picture of the current published work.

A good way of starting a literature review is to find recently published articles or reviews relevant to your research, which will provide a guide to current thinking and sources of references, bearing in mind the results of the research are often published many months after the research was completed. References obtained from a relevant book may be useful but out-of-date.

Whilst a thorough review of the literature is essential preparation for any study, it should be borne in mind that publication of research findings is no guarantee that the research was of a high standard. You should check carefully the sources of your references and should develop your own review and appraisal skills.

Libraries

The most obvious place to start searching for literature is a library. Many hospitals have their own library and may sometimes have access to a University or College library. If you are not familiar with using the literature-searching facilities of a library, the librarian will provide help and advice on how to make the best use of them. If the library does not stock the journal you are looking for, an article can usually be obtained using the inter-library loan scheme. However, this service often incurs a small charge unless you are registered as a student.

Carrying out a Literature Search

There are many ways to search published literature, of which the following three are described below:

- Local access computer search of CD-ROM databases
- Manual searching through journals
- The Internet.

Local Access Computer Search of CD-ROM Databases

Many libraries have CD-ROM databases such as MEDLINE (see below) which are simple to use, and you can do the searches yourself. Before you start searching the databases, you need to choose the keywords you are going to use. If you are unsure of what keywords to use, find recent relevant articles and note the ones that they have used. You should not restrict yourself to one database as you may miss relevant and interesting journals.

Some of the more commonly available CD-ROM databases are:

- **MEDLINE**

  (The printed version is Index Medicus.) This is a major international database covering medicine, dentistry, nursing and veterinary medicine, and pre-clinical sciences such as microbiology, biochemistry and physiology. It contains references to over 3,000 journals and selected conference proceedings. It holds information from 1966 onwards and is updated monthly.

- **CINAHL** (Current Index to Nursing and Allied Health Literature)

  This covers journals from 1983 onwards and is updated monthly. It includes journals covering nursing, physiotherapy, occupational therapy and other allied health disciplines.

- **The Cochrane Library**

  This is a regularly updated electronic library providing evidence for informed health care decision-making. It is recognised worldwide as the most comprehensive source of evidence on health care. Cochrane reviews are of randomised controlled trials published in journals, conference proceeding reports and many other sources and evidence is included or excluded on the basis of explicit quality criteria to minimise bias. (For more information see the Cochrane Web site: http://www.hcn.net.au/cochrane/info.htm.)

- **EMBASE**

  (The printed version is Excerpta Medica.) This provides bibliographic information for more than 3,800 international health care and biomedical journals, indexing from 1980. The coverage includes drugs and toxicology, clinical medicine, basic biological sciences, health affairs, pharmacy, nursing and dentistry.

- **British Nursing Index (BNI)**

  This consolidates the Nursing Bibliography, RCN Nurse ROM and the Nursing and Midwifery Index. It includes over 220 health related journals from 1994 onwards. It covers predominantly English journals on nursing and midwifery and is aimed at nurses, midwives, health visitors and the allied professions.

- **HealthSTAR (formerly known as Health PLAN)**

  This covers non-clinical aspects of health care such as administration, planning, finance, management and related areas. Coverage is from 1975 and includes approximately 840,000 citations supplied by US National Library of Medicine and the American Hospital Association.

Manual Searching through Journals

If you are looking for general information concerning your subject, a relevant book will be adequate. However, if you require more detailed and up-to-date information, you should look for periodical (journal) articles on your topic of interest. For this, you can use CD-ROM databases (as described above), or printed indices and abstracts in the library.

- **Indices** contain bibliographic references, e.g. author, article title and periodical title.

- **Abstracts** are the same as indices but also include a summary of the article.

You can search through abstracts and indices using subject subdivision (keywords) or by author. Alternatively, you could find a journal concerning your topic and search for articles of interest in the issues available. References from such articles may provide other sources of information.

Internet

This is becoming increasingly important to the researcher. The World Wide Web (also known as 'the Web', 'W3' or 'WWW') comprises a universe of all network-accessible information which can be delivered to your desktop.

The Web began in March 1989 when Tim Berners-Lee (then at CERN, the European high energy physics laboratory) released the initial software as a means of moving data and research ideas effectively throughout the organisation. It was quickly taken up and there are now more than 100 countries involved.

How Do I Get Connected ?

Almost any computer can access the Web; all that is normally required is a network card or, if you have a single or stand-alone personal computer (PC), you will need a modem. You will need to acquire some software called a 'browser' - a programme you load on your PC which decodes and displays the information requested. The Web is an example of client and server, where you are the client and the server (which holds the information) is remote (often in another country). You request information using your browser and it is delivered from the server to your desktop. The two most common browsers are Microsoft's Internet Explorer and Netscape. Internet Explorer is freeware (i.e. available at no cost) and is being developed to integrate into Microsoft's other suite of products.

Which Site Should I Connect to ?

There are literally tens of thousands of Web servers. To find the one that you need, you require a standard method of access, and, just as you have a specific home address, so do servers. They are called Uniform Resource Locators (URLs) and are found increasingly in books, magazines, newspapers and even roadside advertising; they are simply pointers to where information resides. URLs usually start with the letters 'http', which stands for HyperText Transfer Protocol; this is the main protocol which connects the client to the server. A typical URL might be:

http://www.man.ac.uk

Typing the above into your browser will request information from the University of Manchester's homepage. Note that URLs are letter and case sensitive; if you copy them from newspapers or journals, be very careful. The above URL will work; the one below will not.

http://WWW.man.ac.uk

How Do I Navigate through the Information ?

The Web relies on hypertext, or, more properly, hypermedia, to navigate through and across documents. Here, significant words will be in a different colour and clicking on that item will invoke a new URL, i.e. a pointer to further information on that topic. By this method, unlike a book, readers will 'filter' through information in different ways, reflecting their varying backgrounds and interests.

How Do I Search for Information ?

If you wish to find information on, say, hypertension and you don't have a URL, it is probably easiest to use a 'search engine'. These are pieces of software that you can access from your browser. In the search engine you type in the search item, say, 'hypertension', and it will roam the Web and return all the sites ('hits') that it has found to you in hypertext format, i.e. you will only have to click to go to that site. Here are the URLs of a few useful search engines:

Alta Vista: http://www.altavista.digital.com
Yahoo: http://www.yahoo.com
Lycos: http://fuzine.mt.cs.cmu.edu/mlm/lycos-home.html
Infoseek: http://www2.infoseek.com

What Is on the Web ?

There is information on practically everything. However, it may often appear anarchic as no special permission is required to publish on the Web. Most people use a feature on their browsers called 'bookmarks' to remember their favourite URLs. All information delivered to your desktop, including images, can be printed using your local printer. You should follow the normal rules for copyright material and provide appropriate references.

There is a large repertoire of sites which cater for medicine. Table 1 gives some sites of particular interest.

The cost of accessing the Web depends on where you are trying to access it from. Some organisations (e.g. Universities) do not charge individual users for using the Web, although the organisation may have to pay a fee. If you are accessing the Web via a standalone PC and modem then the charge will be approximately that of a telephone call, i.e. the time connected to the Internet per minute will equal the same as the rate for a telephone call per minute.

OMIM (On-line Mendelian Inheritance in Man): **http://www3.ncbi.nlm.nih.gov/Omim** This site is devoted to Mendelian Inherited conditions - you simply type in the search string, say, 'Marfans Syndrome', and it will return an essay giving the latest information on that topic. These documents are regularly updated.
PubMed: **http://www3.ncbi.nlm.nih.gov/PubMed** This is a free MEDLINE service from the National Library of Medicine.
The Virtual Hospital: **http://indy.radiology.uiowa.edu/VirtualHospital.html** This site is based at the University of Iowa and embraces a large collection of clinical departments.
Webpath **http://www-medlib.med.utah.edu/WebPath/webpath.html** This site has over 1,800 images together with text and tutorials demonstrating gross and microscopic pathologic findings associated with disease states.
National Cancer Institute (NCI): **http://www.nci.nih.gov/** This is a prime site for oncology and is based at the National Institute of Health in Bethesda, Maryland.
Society for the Internet in Medicine: **http://www.mednet.org.uk/mednet** This was formed to promote the education of the public and of the medical community in the application of the Internet in medical sciences.
Telescan: **http://telescan.nki.nl/** The Telematics Services in Cancer site is the first European Internet service for cancer research, treatment and education.
It is worth enquiring if your professional body or area of expertise has a Web site. There is an e-mail network specifically for physiotherapists, which is also a useful source of Web site addresses.

Table 1: Useful Internet sites

Accessing Expertise

It is essential to discuss your research ideas with colleagues, experts in the field and experienced researchers. There may be others in different professions with similar interests whose advice may be valuable. There may also be Support Units available in your region which can provide advice on the development of your project. These may have statisticians, health economists and others who will help in your research design and application for funding. It is essential to obtain advice from a statistician on all aspects of data collection and analysis.

Prior to any discussions, you should prepare an outline of your proposed research (see below). If you are not familiar to your contact, it may be appropriate to include a one-page summary of your curriculum vitae (CV), and the meeting is likely to be more fruitful if your research outline and a covering letter are sent well in advance.

The outline should contain the following:

- Research question
- Brief literature review
- Aim
- Outcomes
- Proposed methods.

Choosing an Appropriate Research Methodology

Having reviewed the literature, sought appropriate advice and refined your research idea, you will need to consider which research methodology to adopt. The methodology that you select should be the one which is the most effective to collect accurate data to answer your research question or test your hypothesis.

Research studies may be either quantitative or qualitative; the characteristics of these differing approaches are compared in Table 2. It is possible to use both in a research project.

Quantitative Methods

A vital part of the research process is the gathering of information. In quantitative research, this information takes the form of measurements or counts which are amenable to statistical analysis.

A scientific premise exists when a phenomenon can be measured and, if it can be measured, it can also be understood. Quantitative research therefore deals with quantities, measurements and numbers which are analysed by manipulation of those values by suitable statistical techniques in order that the strength of measured effects, comparisons, differences, trends and associations are known (Currier, 1990).

The entire process of quantitative research follows standard procedures, methods, forms of data analysis, and reporting of the outcomes of research. This standardisation of the process of enquiry maximises objectivity in research; methods can be replicated, controversial results checked by other workers and fraudulent activities minimised.

Qualitative Methods

Qualitative research is more than just non-numerical research, it has been described as '*the interpretative study of a specified issue or problem in which the researcher is central to the sense that is made*' (Bannister et al., 1994). This type of research offers insights and understanding of participants unobtainable by quantitative means. It aims to study things in their natural settings and to collect naturally occurring data (Bowling, 1997) and describes in words rather than numbers the qualities of social phenomena through observation. Qualitative methods include structured and unstructured interviews, group interviews and focus groups.

Question	Quantitative	Qualitative
What is the nature of reality?	Reality is objective and singular, separate from the researcher.	Reality is subjective and multiple, as seen by participants in the study.
What is the relationship of the researcher to what is being researched?	Researcher is independent from what is being researched.	Researcher interacts with what is being researched.
What is the relationship between facts and values?	Facts are value-free and unbiased.	Facts are value-laden and biased.
What is the language of research?	Formal	Informal
What is the process of research?	Deductive	Inductive
	Cause and effect	Mutual simultaneous shaping of factors
	Static design – categories isolated before the study	Emerging design – categories identified during research process
	Context-free	Context-bound
	Generalisations leading to prediction, explanation and understanding	Patterns and theories developed for understanding
	Accurate and reliable through validity and reliability	Accurate and reliable through verification

Table 2: Characteristics of quantitative and qualitative research

Statistics and Health Economics

It is important that the statistical techniques that you apply to your proposed research project are sound in order to ensure that the results of your research are valid. Similarly, it is important that the costs and benefits of the research are taken into consideration to enable comparison to other methods of treatment.

Statistics

The statistical content of a research project is often the most rigorously reviewed element of papers, reports and presentations of the study findings. Many researchers erroneously believe that statistical advice is necessary only at the stage of analysing the data obtained from their study. In fact, statistical concepts need to be considered even at the planning stage of a project. Errors made at the start of a study cannot be rectified by the use of even the most sophisticated of statistical methods.

Discussing your project with a statistician will enable you to design the study and the instruments that you will use to collect the data in the most effective way. They can give advice on the techniques for data collection, analysis and methods and style of reporting, which will enable you to communicate your results effectively. A research proposal which is not statistically valid is unlikely to be recommended for funding by reviewers.

Statistical advice is available to many researchers through Regional Research Support Units. These Units are often located in a University or Trust and are funded through the Regional Office's R&D Directorate to provide advice to all researchers, particularly those in smaller Trusts and the community care sector. The Units provide a range of statistical support as outlined below.

- **Study design** - A variety of different designs are used in both clinical trials and surveys. Consideration of the various options available can often help to clarify achievable study objectives, and the statistical implications of those options can be discussed.
- **Sample selection** - Selecting subjects for studies, particularly surveys, can be more complex than it first appears. Is a simple random sample sufficient or should stratification be used to ensure that important subgroups are adequately represented in the sample?
- **Randomisation** - In clinical trials, patients have to be allocated

appropriately to the test treatments. Advice can be given on how to prepare random allocation schedules.

- **Measures** - Different types of measures have different statistical properties. Often a simple amendment to a measure can produce a substantial improvement in the power or sensitivity of the study.
- **Data management** advice on the structure of databases and spreadsheets. Many research projects encounter unnecessary delays at the analysis stage because inadequate attention has been given to problems such as handling quantitative data and developing appropriate coding schemes for quantitative measures.
- **Data analysis** - With desktop PCs and Windows-based statistical packages, most researchers can complete at least the basic analysis of their data themselves. The Support Units can offer advice on choice of statistical package and can provide appropriate levels of supervision during the data analysis.
- **Presentation and dissemination** - Even the most sophisticated and brilliant statistical analysis will count for little if it cannot be understood. Advice is available on presenting the results of a study. The inference drawn from analyses can also be evaluated, to ensure that the conclusions drawn are truly substantiated by the statistical results.

Statistics Units provide advice when applying for funding and ethical approval. Many of these applications require some sort of formal statistical input; without this, applications to funders are unlikely to be successful.

Health Economics – What Is It and Why Is It Important?

Health economics is the study of how scarce health resources such as medical staff and drugs can be used efficiently to provide the maximum gain in health status for a given cost. Using a resource such as a doctor to provide care to one set of patients is to forego the benefit the doctor would provide to another set. Therefore, the management of these scarce resources within the NHS requires the estimation of the costs and benefits of alternative treatments and programmes of care. These benefits may be in terms of a patient's perceived valuation of different health states or attributes of care delivery (cost utility analysis), monetary valuation of benefits (cost benefit analysis) or changes in natural physical units of health, such as decreases in blood pressure (cost-effectiveness analysis).

Rational decisions as to which programme of care should be funded can be made by comparing the cost-to-benefit ratios of alternatives being evaluated. One of the simplest forms of economic evaluation is to compare the costs of a health care programme with its consequences, which may be multidimensional, e.g. fundholding may result in a reduction in GP prescribing but an increase in referrals. Whilst this does not easily translate into a cost-effectiveness ratio, it still enables decision-makers to understand the consequences and trade-offs of implementing change. Economic evaluations may be conducted alongside any type of study design, whether it be randomised controlled trials or cohort studies.

Many researchers can obtain advice on health economics from the Regional R&D Support Units.

References

Avis, M. Reading Research Critically I: An Introduction to Appraisal: Designs and Objectives. Journal of Clinical Nursing. 1994, 3, 227-234

Avis, M. Reading Research Critically II: An Introduction to Appraisal: Assessing the Evidence. Journal of Clinical Nursing. 1994, 3, 271-277

Bannister, P, Burman, E, Parker, I, Taylor, M & Tindall, C. Qualitative Methods in Psychology: A Research Guide. Buckingham. Open University Press 1994

Bland, M. An Introduction to Medical Statistics (2nd ed.). Oxford University Press 1995

Bowling, A. Research Methods in Health: Investigating Health and Health Services. Open University Press 1997

Currier, DP. Elements of Research in Physical Therapy (3rd ed.). Baltimore. Williams and Wilkins 1990

Fowkes, FGR & Fulton, PM. Critical Appraisal of Published Research: Introduction Guidelines. British Medical Journal. 1991, 302, 1136-1140

Goodman, C. Literature Searching and Evidence Interpretation for Assessing Healthcare Practices. Stockholm. The Swedish Council on Health Technology Assessment 1996

Greenhalgh, T. How to Read a Paper: The Basics of Evidence-Based Medicine. British Medical Journal Publishing Group 1997

Hicks, CM. Research for Physiotherapy: Project Design and Analysis. Edinburgh. Churchill Livingstone 1995

Lockett, T. Health Economics for the Uninitiated. Abingdon. Radcliffe 1996

Oldham, J. Statistical Tests (Part 1): Descriptive Statistics. Nursing Standard. 1993, Vol. 7, 43, pp. 30-35

Oldham, J. Statistical Tests (Part 2): Parametric Tests. Nursing Standard. 1993,

Vol. 7, 44, pp. 28-30

Oldham, J. Statistical Tests (Part 3): Non-Parametric Tests. Nursing Standard. 1993, Vol. 7, 45, pp. 28-30

Roe, B. Undertaking a Critical Review of the Literature. Nurse Researcher. 1993, 1(1), 31-42

Checklist

1. Have you carried out a literature review?
2. Have you consulted with colleagues, experts in the field and experienced researchers?
3. Have you consulted a statistician?
4. Do you have an outline research proposal?
5. Have you decided on a research methodology?

4) WRITING A RESEARCH PROPOSAL

- Research protocol
- Resources
- Evaluating research

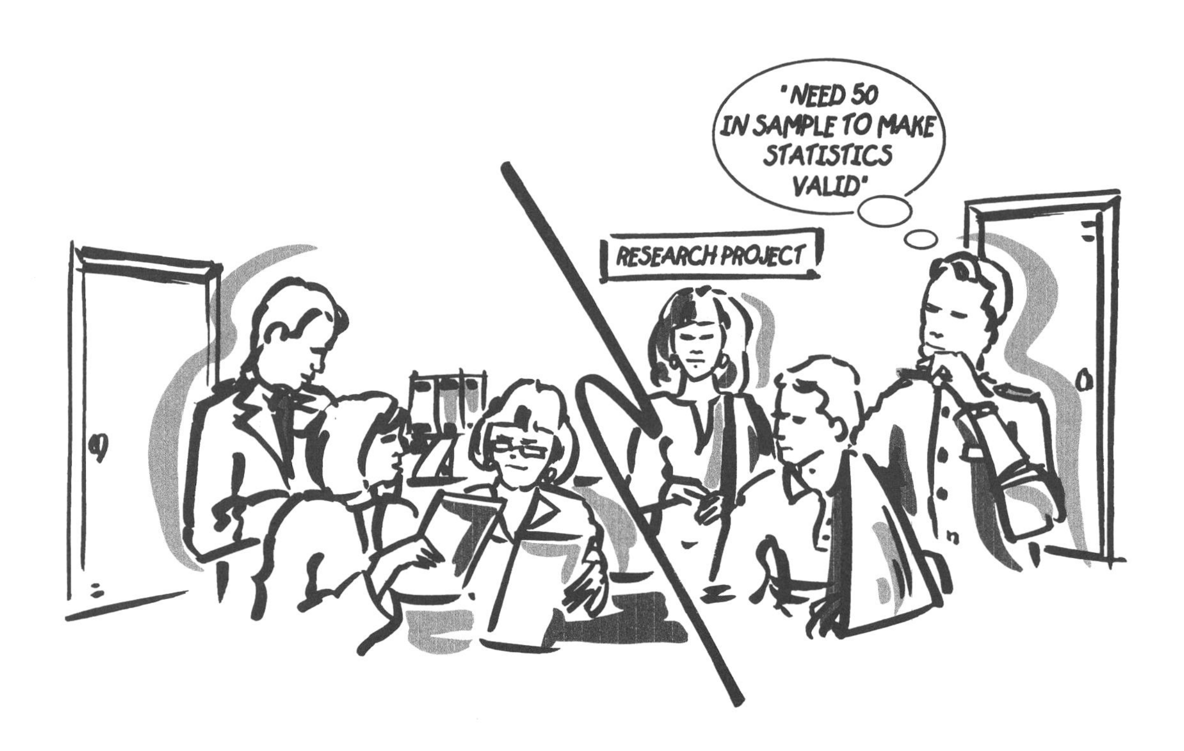

The documentation of all the component parts and stages of the research process is called the research protocol. The protocol is a structured description of the research and should cover all elements of the proposed study.
A protocol fulfils a number of important functions:

- It forms the accurate record of the intentions of the researcher.
- It is an aid to the planning of the project.
- It forms the basis of information when applying for funding, Ethics Committee approval and any other bodies' permission which may be required before commencing the study.
- It forms part of any contract documentation and is therefore a legal document.

The protocol should be appropriately worded according to its intended readership and purpose. Applications for higher and research degrees require a protocol to provide a reasoned argument to justify the study, detail how it will be carried out and indicate the likely outcomes.
It is unlikely that any single protocol will be suitable for all applications, although all protocols will contain similar information. It is important to ensure that each is suitable for its intended purpose, i.e. in the correct format or on an appropriate form.
The contents of a typical research protocol are given below.

Protocol Contents

Title

This should be brief and informative, and clearly identify the project and its objectives.

Summary or Abstract

This should be a synopsis of the study, ideally of around 250 words, stating the purpose of the research. It should describe the study design and methods of data collection, and outline the expected findings. This may take the form of a list of the main components of the protocol, each with an accompanying note. The name of the principal researcher should be included, along with qualifications and relevant experience. The names of other contributors to the study must always be included. Include the contact address and telephone number of the principal researcher. Note that a full CV will be required in some circumstances and it is good practice to update your CV regularly.

Background and Rationale of Your Study

Describe succinctly the health issue to be addressed. This may include the prevalence of a problem, identification of a patient group, the burden of care provision on a particular service, perceived etiological factors, the implications of continuing care, etc. The main clinical and conceptual issues should be stated clearly, and where the proposed research fits into the framework of existing research, knowledge or practice. A brief literature review should be included and the references appended in full at the end of the document.

Aims and Objectives

The broad aims of the study should be stated; the primary (and secondary, if appropriate) objectives should be detailed. This might include the expected benefits of the study and how the results will be taken forward.

Experimental Design and Methods

> Advice from a statistician and health economist at the design stage of your project is vital.

This section of the protocol should provide details of the study design and how the objectives of the study will be met (or how the hypothesis will be tested). It should include information on:

- The number of subjects to be studied - A statistician should be consulted to provide a 'power calculation' to show that an appropriate number of subjects will be recruited to the study.
- How the subjects will be selected (sampling methods)
- Patient inclusion and exclusion criteria
- How the patients will be recruited and the information they will be given to allow them to decide whether to participate in the research
- The type of study proposed, whether quantitative (e.g. blind/double or blind randomised) or qualitative (e.g. participant or non-participant observation, or focus groups)
- The procedures or interventions to be used on subjects (e.g. blood samples, tests and drugs) including any risk issues
- The data to be collected and how they will be coded
- The methods to be used to collect data:
    - ♦ The instruments (e.g. questionnaires and measuring devices) should be described, together with the rationale for their use.

- ♦ Issues of validity and reliability should be addressed. References to the existing literature or previous pilot studies are appropriate.
- The methods of data analysis - For both qualitative and quantitative studies, it is necessary to seek advice. Advice can be obtained from a statistician or someone who has experience in qualitative research.

Ethical Considerations

All research which involves patients or their records will need approval from the Local Research Ethics Committee (LREC). This approval is primarily concerned with the welfare and dignity of the participants of any research project, together with the validity of the study. The LREC ensures that individuals are not tested unnecessarily and are not misinformed or ill-treated.

It also seeks to ensure compliance with regulations and provides researchers with some protection in the event of legal claims. This topic is fully covered in Chapter 5.

Intellectual Property

There is a great pressure to publish the findings of your research as soon as it is complete. If, however, your work has produced some new or novel ideas, you should make an assessment of their suitability for further exploitation and development, especially if there is potential for commercial use. The tangible output of any intellectual activity can legitimately be described as intellectual property (IP). The processes of protection and exploitation of IP are complementary to the normal processes of dissemination. Carried out effectively, IP exploitation may provide further resources for the NHS, for both patients and research. It is a complex subject and, if you think you have an idea suitable for development, contact your Trust's R&D office or the Regional Office's R&D Directorate. You must do this before you publish or present your work; once it is in the public domain, most of the exploitation potential has been lost. The NHS has published guidance for researchers and their Trusts in HSC 98 (106).

IP may arise in the form of new drugs but is more likely to be new devices, software, know-how or printed material. It can be protected by patents, design rights or copyright. Some forms of protection (such as copyright) are free, while others (such as patents) are expensive and often take years to realise commercial return. However, the early stages of any protection process are quick and should not delay publication for more than one or two weeks.

The ownership of the intellectual property or copyright of the research should be established at the stage when you set up your funding contract; usually ownership of intellectual property defaults to the sponsor or your employer.

A separate handbook describing in more detail how to protect and manage new ideas and inventions will be available from the same source as this handbook (see back of front cover for details).

Benefits of the Study

The benefits of the study need to be identified. These may be more effective or efficient health care, improved knowledge or the facilitation of further research. Identification of the benefits, especially those pertaining to cost benefits, may require advice from a health economics specialist.

Resources and Costs

You must be careful to assess all the potential costs of your research. There are four broad categories defined by the NHS in Health Service Guidelines (97)32:

- **Infrastructure costs** such as space, your own time and the costs of maintaining the buildings - These costs may be met by your organisation through the NHS R&D Support Funding which it may receive. Your organisation is not obliged to provide you with any new equipment or facilities to carry out your work.
- **R&D costs** - These are the costs of the research itself, and will include new equipment, staff dedicated wholly or in part to the project, and data collection and analysis. These costs are met by the funder of your project.
- **Service Support costs** are the additional patient care costs, e.g. extra blood tests, nursing attention or x-rays. These costs may be met by your organisation through NHS R&D Support Funding or from your project sponsor.
- **Excess Treatment costs** are where patient care costs are in excess of standard treatment costs or will continue after the research has finished. These are funded from the normal contracting arrangements between your Trust and Health Authorities.

Be realistic with your costings as, once the sponsor has awarded you a sum, it will be very difficult to obtain further funds if you have underestimated the costs and this may jeopardise your ability to complete your work. Also, many sponsors have a restriction on the amount of funding which can be vired from one cost heading to another. Ensure that all items (capital and recurrent) are included and can be justified. It is essential to consult your Trust accountant in determining the costs involved in your research. Full costing details will be required in your funding applications and you will require a statement from the Trust giving permission to use organisational resources. This is described in more detail in Chapter 7.

Project Plan and Monitoring

Project planning is an extremely important part of any research project and it is described in more details in Chapter 8.

Development Protocol

The elements and contents of the development protocol are essentially similar to those included in a research protocol (see Chapter 4). Development work will focus on whether the research results will be achieved in a practical setting.

References

Bandolier 36. 1997, 4, 2 February; Pain Relief Unit, The Churchill, Oxford, OX3 7LJ

Currier, DP. Elements of Research in Physical Therapy (3rd ed.). Baltimore. Williams and Wilkins 1990

Drummond, A. Research Methods for Therapists. London. Chapman and Hall 1996

Health Service Circular 98 (106): Policy Framework for the Management of Intellectual Property in the NHS

Health Service Guidelines (97)32: Meeting Patient Care Costs Associated with R&D in the NHS

Luscombe, D & Stonier, P. (eds.). Clinical Research Manual. Haslemere. Euromed Communications 1994

Sources of systematic reviews are:

- The Cochrane Collaboration Centre, Summertown Pavilion, Middle Way, Oxford
- Centre for Reviews and Dissemination, Alcuin College, University of York, York YO1 5DD

Checklist

1. Have all the necessary items been included in the protocol?
2. Was a statistician consulted on experimental design?
3. Have IP rights and copyright of research been established?
4. Has a list of the required resources and costs been made?
5. Have plans for dissemination been made?

5) ETHICAL CONSIDERATIONS

- Role of Ethics Committees
- Application procedure
- Informed consent
- Multi-centre trials

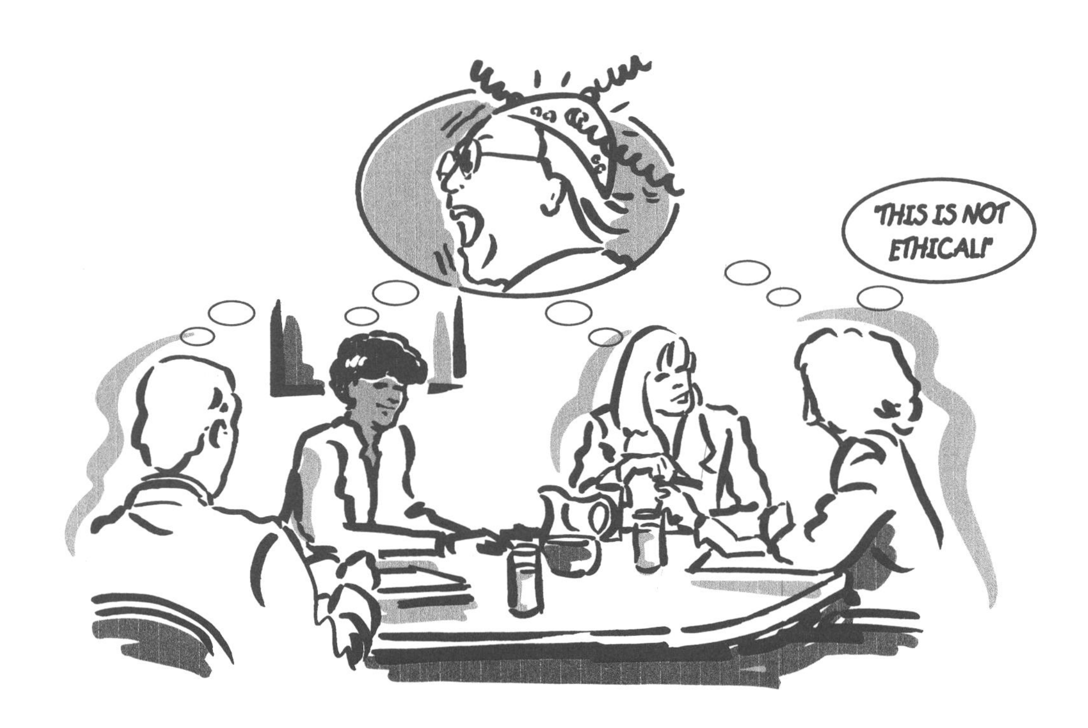

Overview

When planning clinical research, you should always pay careful attention to the ethical issues which may result from your work. Clinical research generally involves the participation of patients, staff, healthy volunteers or students, and ethical and legal issues are therefore likely to be raised. To ensure that patients and others are protected, Local Research Ethics Committees (LRECs), usually administered by Health Authorities, have been put in place, working to nationally published guidelines. LRECs are primarily concerned with the welfare and dignity of the participants of any research project, as well as the validity of the study. The LREC ensures that individuals are not tested unnecessarily and are not misinformed or ill-treated.

If your study involves the participation of students, you may require ethical approval from the institute providing your student population, in addition to approval from your LREC.

Role of the Local Research Ethics Committee

The LRECs are usually organised geographically by health district and their purpose is '*to consider the ethics of proposed research projects which will involve human subjects and which will take place broadly within the NHS*'. They are also concerned with the quality and integrity of a project. The guidelines issued by the Department of Health in Health Service Guideline (91)5 state that any research involving the following requires ethical approval:

- NHS patients (past or present)
- Foetal material and in vitro fertilisation involving NHS patients
- The recently dead, in NHS premises
- Access to records of past or present NHS patients
- The use of, or potential access to, NHS premises or facilities.

Application Procedure

The appropriate LREC should be contacted in the initial stages of protocol development if there is any doubt about whether ethical approval is required. Certain types of research (e.g. laboratory-based studies) may be exempt from the need for LREC approval, but you should check on this before starting work. You may find that both your employing organisation and your research sponsor require written ethical approval or a waiver from the requirements of ethical approval.

Early contact with the administrator of the LREC is also advised in order to check the dates of meetings and submission dates.

In order to gain ethical approval, an application form should be completed; the form can be obtained from the secretary to the Ethics Committee. Forms may vary between LRECs, but most will have questions which fall into the following categories:

- Project title
- Names and details of investigators
- Study objectives
- Outline of study design
- Scientific background to study
- Recruitment details
- Tests, instruments, drugs and devices to be used
- GPs' consent
- Potential discomfort and risks to subjects
- Informed consent (consent form and patient information sheet)
- Indemnity from drug or equipment suppliers (see Chapter 6 for more details)
- Cost and sponsor payment details

When applying for ethical approval, it is important to remember that some members of the Ethics Committee are lay members and there may not be a member who is a specialist in your area of research. Therefore, it is necessary for the document to be non-technical and readable. When assessing the application the LREC will look for the following points:

- Any possible effects on the individuals' health
- The scientific merit of the project
- Possible hazards and proposed ways of handling them
- Expected degree of discomfort or distress for the participants
- Adequate supervision from suitably qualified and experienced personnel
- Inducements to be offered to patients or the investigators
- Suitability of the information sheet

- Procedures for obtaining consent from the subjects or, where necessary, their parents or guardians
- Measures in place to ensure subject confidentiality.

If you do receive ethical approval, this does not give authorisation for the project to proceed. The project still requires approval from the organisation(s) in which you intend to carry out the research.

Points to Consider

Recruitment

Potential subjects should never be coerced or made to take part in a study against their will. The investigators should emphasise the fact that participation is voluntary and that participants can withdraw from the study at any time without detriment to their treatment. It is the responsibility of the researchers to ensure that the participants have no contra-indications to the study.

Obtaining Participant Consent

Written informed consent is required from all participants and the LREC will want evidence that a volunteer will be given enough information to provide this. Both a written and verbal explanation of the study is usually required before the participant signs the consent form. Some LRECs have a standard consent form which should be used in conjunction with the information sheet.

Items to include on the patient information sheet are:

- The purpose of the study
- Details of the procedures involved and what is required of the participants
- Length of the study
- Any effect on patients' treatment by participating in the trial
- Any potential harmful effects or discomfort they may have as well as any potential benefits
- Assurance of confidentiality and compliance with the Data Protection Act

Tips on designing an information sheet are:

- Use short sentences
- Avoid jargon and medical terms or explain such language when used

- Wherever possible, use lists or bullet points instead of paragraphs
- Use subheadings
- Use a minimum of 12-point font size
- Make sure it is easy to read, several versions in different languages may be needed

It may be appropriate to use a question-and-answer format (Wager et al., 1995).

Some studies require the use of participants who may find it difficult or impossible to give informed consent, e.g. the elderly or children. In these cases, the LREC will seek the appropriate specialist advice.

Multi-Centre Trials

Multi-Centre Research Ethics Committees (MRECs) have been set up to give approval to studies that are multi-centre, spread over regions, and involve five or more LRECs. If an MREC approves a multi-centre study, the application must still be submitted to the LRECs for all the research sites. The LREC may then approve or reject the study, but on local study groups only.

For further details about the MREC, contact the appropriate MREC administrator (their address can be obtained from your LREC office).

Research on Animals

A Home Office licence is required for any experiments involving animals. Your Trust may have its own rules and regulations about the conduct of animal work on its premises.

References

Health Service Guidelines (91)5 ('the Red Book')

Health Service Guidelines (97)23: Ethics Committee Review of Multi-Centre Research

Usherwood, T. Introduction to Project Management in Health Research: A Guide For New Researchers. Buckingham, Philadelphia. Open University Press 1996

Wager, E, Tooley, PJH , Emanuel, MB & Wood, S. 1995 How to Do it: Get Patients' Consent to Enter Clinical Trials. British Medical Journal. 31, 734-737.

Checklist

1. Contact the LREC to check if ethical approval is needed and, if so, to obtain an application form.
2. Is there a standard consent form or do you need to design one?
3. Have you a patient/volunteer information sheet? If you are using both types of participant, you may be required to have two sets of information sheets and consent forms.
4. Are all your documents easy to read?
5. Do you have all the documents required by the LREC/MREC?

6) CLINICAL INDEMNITY AND LEGAL ISSUES

- Clinical risks
- Research contracts

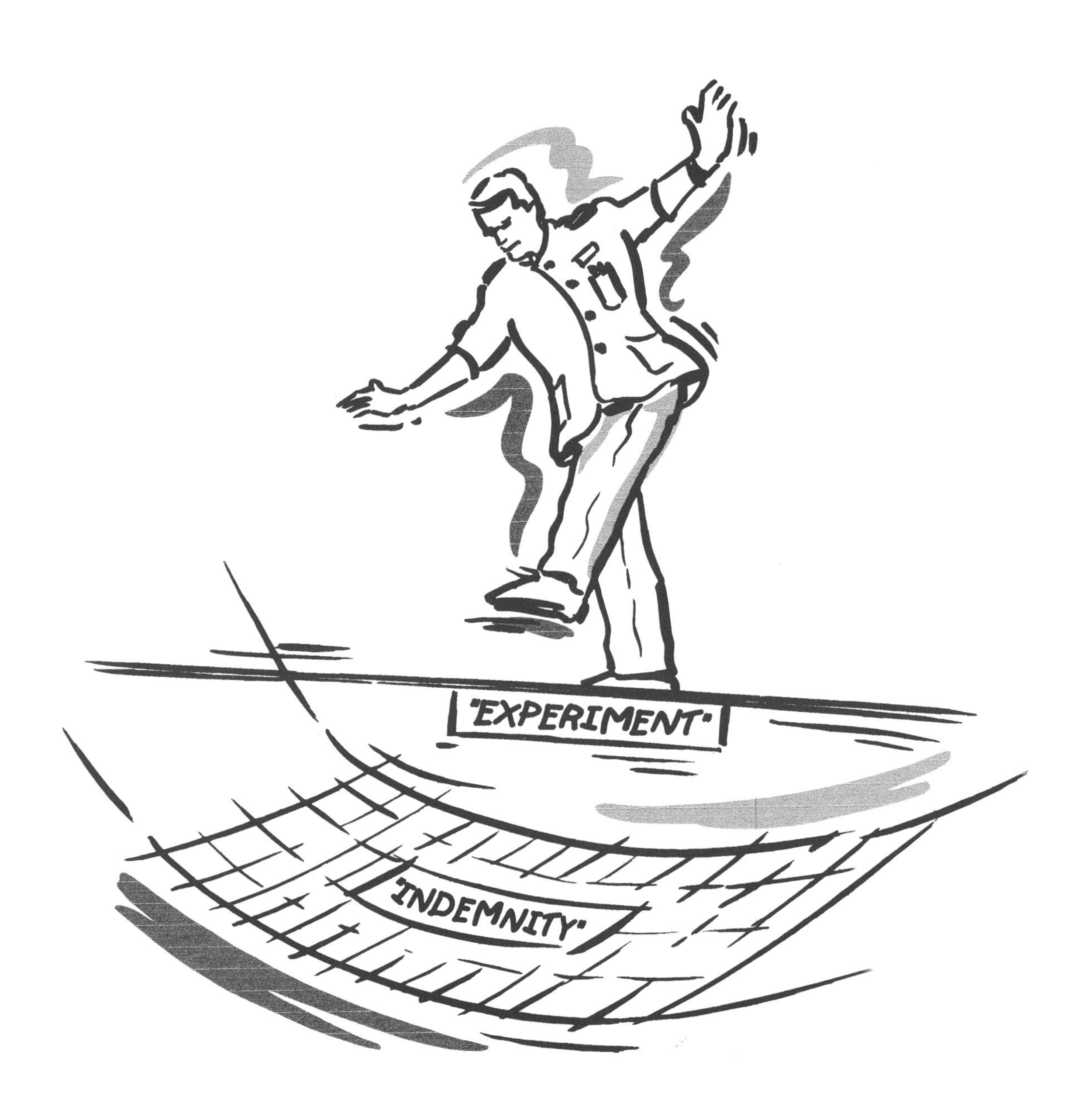

Clinical Risks

All health care work which involves treating patients carries some degree of risk, however slight. Accordingly, hospitals and doctors hold 'clinical negligence insurance' which ensures that, in the quite rare instances that patients do come to harm, the patients have means of getting compensation which does not require wilful fault to be proven. In the same way, clinical research will inevitably carry some risk. The risks to patients can be minimised by well-designed research protocols which have been approved by the Research Ethics Committee.

It is important therefore that you talk to the appropriate person in your organisation to ensure that the study you intend to carry out is covered by the appropriate insurance. In the vast majority of cases - that is, in all NHS Trusts - the Trust's insurance **will** cover you for your research.

There is, however, an important distinction where the research is sponsored by a commercial company. In this case, the sponsoring company must provide your Trust with a 'clinical indemnity form'. This gives the Trust indemnity against the drug or device that you are testing or trialling being inherently faulty.

The NHS has published some quite clear guidance on clinical indemnity in Health Service Guideline (97)48. It also provides a standard clinical indemnity form for you to use. The indemnity form is a legal document and you should make sure that it is signed by the appropriate manager in your Trust (frequently the Chief Executive, Finance Director or R&D Director).

Your Trust should always be aware of research you are intending to pursue and any major changes which occur during the life of your project .

> You should NOT enter into any agreement with a commercial organisation to undertake or support any R&D activities without prior written permission from your Trust.

Contracts for Research

Many research sponsors will require a contract between the researcher, employing organisation and sponsor. In the case of funding from the Department of Health or other agencies, the contract is usually straightforward and is, in simple terms, a method of transferring the funding from the sponsor to the researcher in a structured way, which sets out some simple terms and conditions with which the researcher must comply to receive funding. Most particularly, producing an end-of-project report is usually required, otherwise the final payment is withheld.

In the case of the major charities, the contract will deal with more complex issues, such as 'intellectual property' and 'the right to publish'. If you do not fully understand the contract, always refer back to the sponsor in the first case. It may also be that your Trust has someone who specifically looks after these areas; this person is a valuable source of information.

Please remember that the contract is a legal document and it must be signed by a person within your organisation who has the authority to sign contracts (check with your R&D office).

The insurance and legal aspects of your project should be completed before you apply to your sponsor. To avoid delay, you should submit your indemnity form and contract documents to the appropriate person, who will check and sign them. Occasionally, complex contracts may need to be checked by your organisation's legal adviser. There may be a cost for this and you should ensure that you have the funding available to meet these costs.

Checklist

1. Is your project covered by your Trust's insurance or other clinical risk insurance?
2. Do you need a clinical indemnity form?
3. Do you have an appropriate contract?
4. Has the contract been signed by someone who has the authority to do so?

References

NHS Executive 1996, NHS Indemnity – Arrangements for Clinical Negligence Claims in the NHS

HSG (96) 48, NHS indemnity arrangements for handling clinical negligence claims against NHS staff.

7) FUNDING THE COSTS OF YOUR RESEARCH

- Grant applications
- NHS funding
- National funding

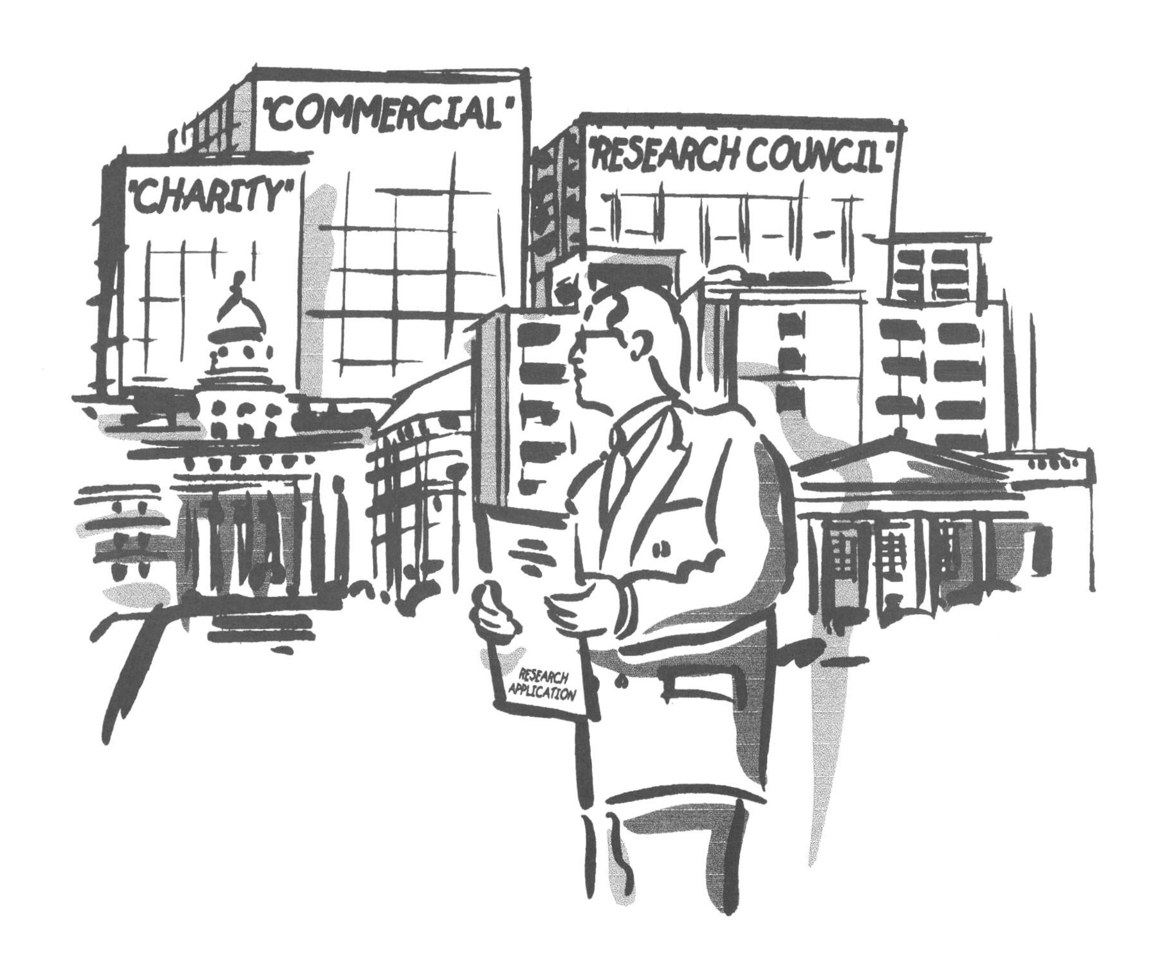

All research has a cost, whether it is of your own time to write your proposals; of employing someone to collect data; or of the consumables used. You must be clear about these potential costs and have proposals to fund them.

There are many sources of external funding, including the NHS, which provides funding for research which is relevant to the NHS and meets defined quality standards. Most research sponsors, including the NHS, research councils and charities, use a system of 'peer review' to assess requests for funding, as a means of quality control and duplication. The NHS also provides funding for the infrastructure to support research; this is termed NHS R&D Support Funding and it is allocated to Trusts in a national **competitive** exercise on either an annual or four-year cycle.

Many worthwhile research studies can be undertaken without the need for external financial support. Small self-funded projects and pilot studies can often provide the basis for subsequent successful grant applications. These **unfunded** studies should still be capable of meeting the same minimum quality standards that are required of externally assessed research.

Submitting Grant Applications

The research priorities and interests of the many funding bodies and agencies vary considerably, according to the aims and objectives of the organisation concerned.

The amounts of funding are variable and some sponsors will only provide a proportion of the funds required. In this case you, as the **researcher**, will be responsible for securing the balance from either another sponsor or your Trust, whose agreement to provide the balance of the total funding requirement must be secured before an application for partial funding is submitted. The basis for this principle of partial funding is that the NHS (and its patients) will ultimately derive benefit from the research and therefore should contribute to the costs, i.e. a partnership. These principles are described in Executive Letter (97)77, which describes the various steps that researchers must take to notify their Trusts of new research, and the Trusts approval considerations.

Competition for funds is intense and applications which are well thought out and well written, and which meet the sponsor's criteria, are more likely to be successful. It is advisable to discuss your plans for funding with your potential sponsor in the early planning stages of your study.

It is essential to cost your proposals accurately (see Chapters 4 and 8). All the direct and indirect costs of your project, and any overheads, should be included, as well as the effects or impact on other departments and professions, e.g. pathology or biochemistry laboratory costs, and statistical analysis or computing. You should seek advice from your organisation's accountant.

When applying for funding for research, it is important to follow the procedures set out by the potential sponsor. Funding bodies usually provide information and guidance, and supply standard application forms for completion. The guidelines should be followed exactly and all sections on the form should be completed. It is important to direct applications to the most appropriate organisation. Therefore, prior planning and informal enquiries to the funding bodies are essential.

Trusts are required by Executive Letter (97)77 to have an established channel (e.g. the R&D, or other designated, manager) through which all bids and funding applications are passed for approval, and to maintain a record of all proposed and current research. This aspect is important for insurance compliance, and your Trust's R&D office will also check any contract documents (see Chapter 6). Applications for funds which are to be sent to an external sponsor by e-mail should be agreed with the Trust's R&D manager **before** submission.

Responsibilities for Research Funds

Ensuring proper use of funds is the responsibility of the applicant or lead researcher and it is essential that full records of expenditure are kept. Providers of funds may require regular updates of progress of the study and of expenditure.

Many funding bodies will withhold the final payment until the end-of-project report is submitted and approved. It is the responsibility of the grant holder to ensure that all conditions of the funding are met and to ensure proper use of the funds. It is essential that accounts are kept for inspection if required.

When you intend to spend your grant, it is advisable to discuss this with your organisation's accountant to ensure that you comply with the necessary rules and regulations. Your accountant will also be able to advise on how to arrange the purchases required for the study with the purchasing department, in order to take advantage of any supply contracts which may have been negotiated, and instances where you can reclaim VAT. If your funding is from a recognised charity, you may be able to hold your accounts in an endowment fund and often these will attract interest on any unspent balances.

Sources of Funding

There are many sources of funding and you should seek out the ones most appropriate to your proposed study. You may increase your chances of success if you target more than one source. In this handbook, it is not possible to list all the sponsors, and you can obtain advice from libraries, Trusts' R&D offices, University grants offices and your professional organisation. The Internet is increasingly the most effective source of advice on what funds are available, including foreign sponsors. A list of commonly used Internet addresses and details of the main sources of health services research funding are included in Appendix B.

The National Health Service Funding Schemes

The NHS, through various funding schemes administered by the Regional Offices' R&D departments, provide funding for direct costs of research. There are two main types, reactive and commissioned.

Reactive Funding Schemes

As the name suggests, these schemes are designed to respond to ideas from researchers across a broad spectrum. They do have some specific criteria, e.g. the proposed research should be good quality, multidisciplinary and relevant to the needs of the NHS. The NHS will also fund development proposals to facilitate the experimental introduction of research-based clinical or organisational developments, of proven efficiency, to improve health.

Commissioned R&D

This is research proactively commissioned by the NHS to provide evidence in a number of priority areas which have been agreed nationally or locally after wide consultation. Nationally, ten priority areas have been identified. Each programme is managed on behalf of the NHS by a Regional Office. The programmes are described in Appendix C (please also see page 15).

Other National Funding Sources

Profession-Specific Funds

Each governing body will have details of funding arrangements, e.g. the British Dental Association, College of Optometrists, United Kingdom Pharmacy

Association, Royal Pharmaceutical Society, College of Radiographers, Chartered Society of Physiotherapists, and Society of Chiropodists and Podiatrists.

Research Councils

These bodies tend to fund large-scale multidisciplinary projects, but also make awards for training in research. The contact details are included in Appendix B.

Charitable Trusts and Foundations

Guides to these organisations are widely available and a list is included at the end of this chapter.

European Union Funding

Your Trust or University will have details. Advice is also available from the Regional Office's R&D Directorate, Department of Health's International Division, or the Medical Research Council.

Local Sources

These include your employing Trust, individual departmental budgets, dedicated funds, endowment funds, NHS R&D charities or endowments, and academic institutions and centres.

Industry and Commercial Organisations

These are ready sources of funding, but will often not fund outside specific research areas. They may impose restrictions on your ability to use and publish data and almost certainly will require a contract between your organisation and themselves. There are particular NHS requirements for insurance and costing of commercial research and you should discuss these with your Trust's R&D office in advance.

References

Executive Letter (97)77: Meeting Patient Costs Associated with R&D in the NHS

The Directory of Grant-Making Trusts, published by the Charities Aid Foundation, is available in all major public libraries.

The Guide to Major Grant-Making Trusts, published by the Directory of Social Change (DSC), is available from DSC, Radius Works, Back Lane, London NW3 - telephone number 0171 284 4364.

The Association of Medical Research Charities (AMRC) produces a handbook, which is available from AMRC, 29-35 Farringdon Road, London EC1M 3JB - telephone number 0171 404 64540. Examples of research charities are:

- British Heart Foundation
- Stroke Association
- Wellcome Trust
- International Diabetes Federation/Eli Lilley Fund.

Checklist

1. Have you approached an appropriate funding body?
2. Is the application form completed correctly?
3. Have you obtained the appropriate signatures ?
4. Have you routed your grant application through your Trust's R&D manager?

8) PROJECT MANAGEMENT AND PERFORMANCE

- Time management
- Staffing
- Budgeting

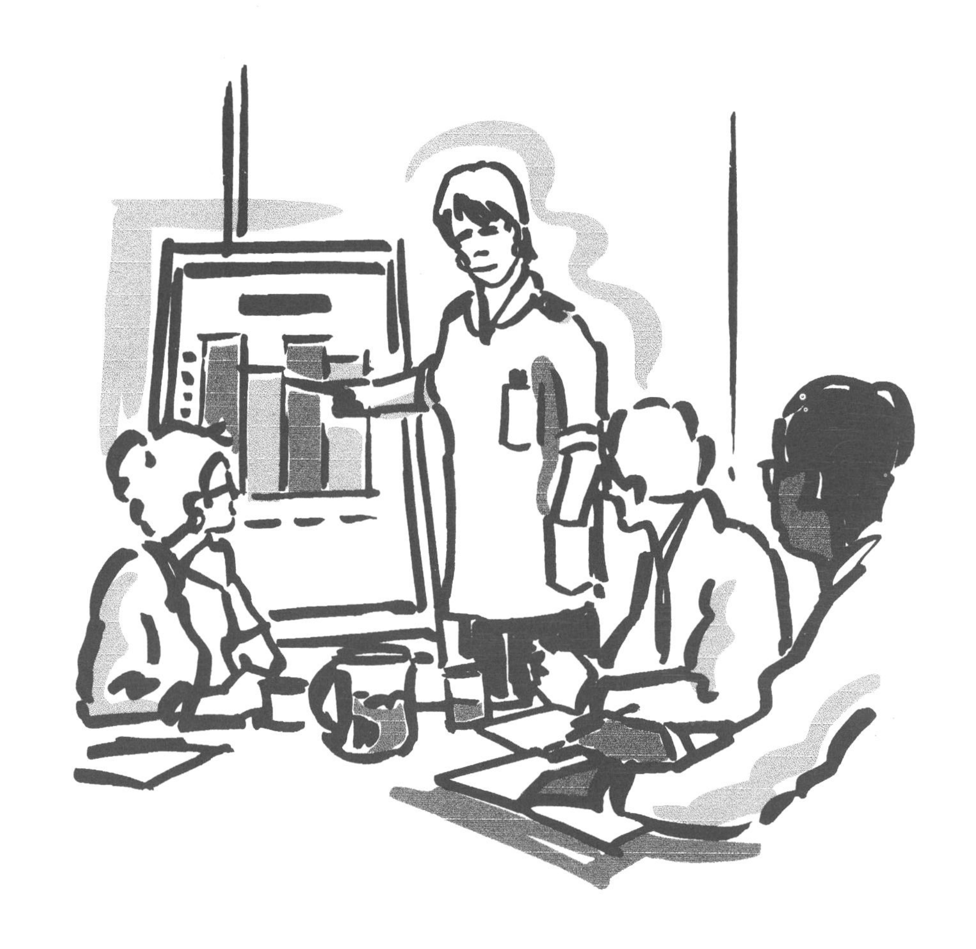

Once you have reached the stage where a research idea has been developed and research objectives decided, you should begin to think about what resources will be needed to carry out the research project and how these are going to be managed. Careful planning of projects will help to make them run more effectively and provide early warning of any problems that may arise.

Resources that might be used in a research project can be categorised as:

- **Time**
- **Staffing**
- **Money (budget).**

Time Management

Organising and managing the time to develop and undertake your research project is an essential element of good research management. Careful time management will help the project to be completed on time and within budget, and will allow its progress to be monitored.

Planning Your Time

It is useful to produce a project timetable and to specify the key milestones that are to be achieved. The following steps will enable you to develop such a timetable to manage and monitor the progress of your project:

- Firstly, list all the activities that need to be undertaken in order to achieve your research objective. This might include only the stages that are to be involved in the research project, such as data collection, entry and analysis, or may be broader and encompass steps such as recruiting staff, obtaining Research Ethics Committee approval or meeting key dates for funding applications.

  As you develop your list of activities, they should be discussed with colleagues who are going to be involved in the research. This is beneficial as it encourages 'brainstorming' and therefore a more exhaustive list is likely to be produced. It also ensures that key milestones and targets are known and agreed at an early stage.

- Having made a list of all the activities to be undertaken, you should estimate the duration of each. You should be realistic and try to anticipate where delays and slippage may occur. Project group members and others should be involved at this stage in order to draw on their experience of how long certain activities will take and to discuss the research schedule.

An example of an activity list, with the expected duration of each stage, is given in Table 3.

Stage	Estimated duration (weeks)
1 Produce questionnaire	9
2 Obtain ethical approval	8
3 Draw sample population	8
4 Recruit patients and obtain consent	16
5 Obtain pre-intervention data	4
6 Collect post-intervention data	4
7 Code and enter data	4
8 Analyse data	4
9 Write up project	8

Table 3: Simple activity and milestone chart

A simple activity list is a useful way of describing how long each stage will take. However, it does not take into consideration that some activities may be able to run in parallel with one another, or may require other steps to be completed before they can commence. This is an important point to consider as it is likely to affect the overall duration of the project. A useful way of illustrating the scheduling of events and the possibility that events will overlap is by using a Gantt chart (see Figure 1).

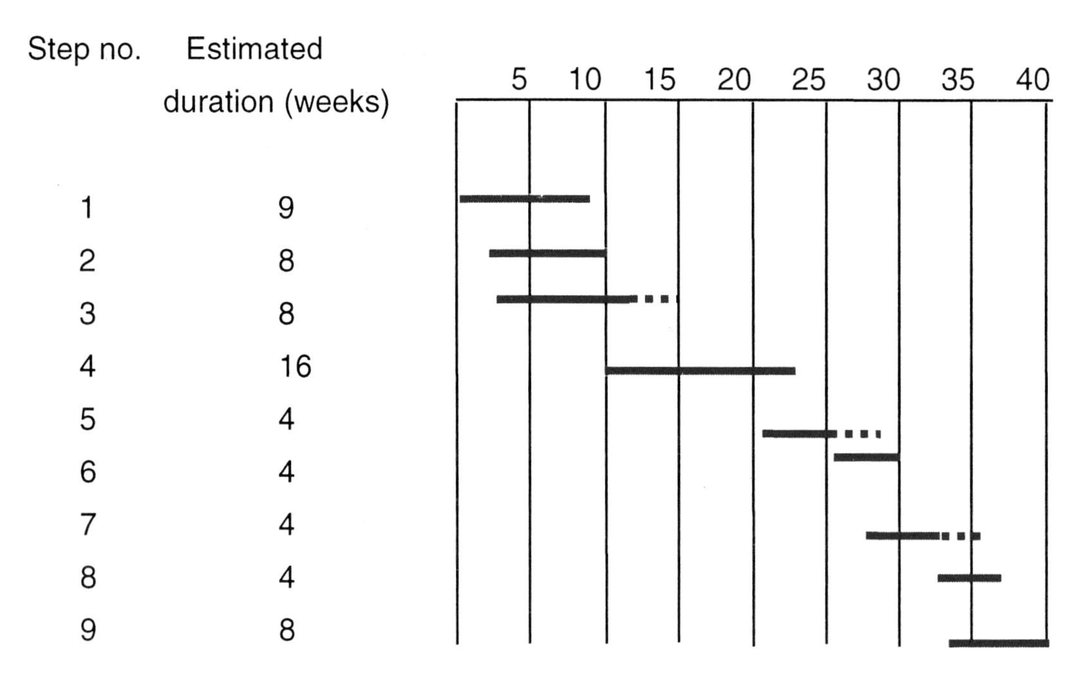

Figure 1: Gantt chart

A Gantt chart lists all the activities that are to be undertaken on the vertical axis and uses a horizontal timescale axis to show how long each will take. Some activities may not start until others have finished (e.g. data analysis - step 8 - cannot start until data collection - step 6 - has been completed), but some activities may overlap or be carried out in parallel with one another (e.g. data entry - step 7 -may start before data collection - step 6 - is complete).

Once produced, a Gantt chart can identify the total duration of the project. The dotted lines on the Gantt chart indicate where an activity may be undertaken later than shown by the solid line. This allows flexibility to be incorporated into the project timetable.

Gantt charts are useful tools to measure the progress of the research project against what has been planned. If your project is taking longer than anticipated, you will need to ensure that your funding will cover the additional time. You may also need to alert the sponsor and agree a new timetable.

Laying out the project in this way enables resources and staff to be scheduled into the project. For example, you can arrange for the statistician, if you are using one, to allow time to analyse your data around week 32. Where slippage has occurred, you can notify the statistician that your data might not be available in week 32. This enables the statistician to work more effectively.

Staffing of Research Projects

Some research projects can be conducted by a single person whilst others may involve many people (some for a defined period to bring a particular skill or area of expertise, e.g. a computer programmer). To produce an activity list, it is likely that a reasonable understanding of the staffing requirements for the execution of the research project will be needed.

In determining the staff required, it is important to think about the number of people you will need, the skills they should have, and the activities they will be involved in. For example, if part of the research project involves taking blood samples for analysis, then you need to determine whether somebody needs to be employed specifically to do this or whether someone who currently undertakes this work could be contracted to do extra samples specifically for the study.

It is good practice to include in the staffing discussions all the people involved in the research, to decide:

- What staffing numbers and skills are required to do the research project?
- Are there suitable people already employed who could do the research?
- Do extra members of staff need to be employed?

If staff need to be employed to work on the project, you must pay careful attention to the amount of funding that will be available, which must include all employment costs, e.g. national insurance, cost of living increases and incremental pay awards. The funding will determine the length of the contract that can be offered and its terms and conditions. A first task is to write an accurate job description, which sets out things such as:

- The job that is required to be done
- Responsibility and accountability arrangements
- Qualifications and experience required of the applicants.

There are many rules and regulations that govern the employment of staff and if you are unfamiliar with them, you should seek help and advice from your organisation's human resources or personnel department.

Budget Management

In your grant application, you will have given a detailed breakdown of the estimated costs of your proposed research project. You may have to provide a spending profile, which will allow the sponsor to make staged payments against the progress of your project. The budget requested in your application may look something like that shown below (Table 4).

Item	Year 1 £	Year 2 £
Staff costs	30,000	15,000
Capital costs		
- computer equipment	2,000	-
Consumables		
- photocopying	150	200
- postage	100	50
Overheads	3,200	3,200
Subtotals	35,450	18,450
TOTAL		**53,900**

Table 4: Budget for research project

Depending upon the scale and complexity of your project, some method of managing the financial aspects of your project is essential, to ensure that you can complete your proposed work. For complex projects, purpose-designed software might be needed, or you may choose to set up a financial spreadsheet in one of the proprietary software packages, e.g. Microsoft Excel. Many projects will be able to be managed with a simple budget plan. An initial task is to list all the activities, with your estimates of the costs and the actual funding received from the sponsor. This check against the funding requested and received is essential as the costs may have risen (or fallen) in the time between your estimate and the receipt of the funding.

Using the list of activities and the funding available, items such as salaries will need to be scheduled on a monthly basis. As expenditure is committed, for example a computer is ordered, it should be recorded against the budget available. When the computer is received and the invoice paid, the amount should be compared against the sum committed, and adjusted if necessary. In this way, you are able to keep an up-to-date account of the budget, commitments and actual expenditure incurred. By monitoring the budget carefully through the duration of the project, you will identify how much money is left, whether it is sufficient to finish the project, and where the money has been spent. Besides being a useful tool in managing your project, the records of expenditure will provide the necessary documentation if your sponsor or Trust wishes to carry out an audit. A simple budget control plan is shown in Table 5, using the example from above.

Date	Item	Budget £	Cost £	Balance £
Salaries				
01.04.98 - 31.03.99	- salaries	30,000	28,000	2,000 less spent than expected
Capital				
30.04.98	- computers	2,000	1,500	
01.06.98	- printers	-	550	
			2050	(50)* spent over budget
Consumables				
01.04.98 - 31.03.99	- photocopying	150	200	(50)* spent over budget
01.04.98 - 31.03.99	- postage	100	120	(20)* spent over budget
Overheads				
01.04.98	- overheads	3,200	3,200	on target
TOTAL		**35,450**	**33,570**	**1,880**

* Using standard accounting notation, overspends are shown in brackets.

Table 5: Budget control chart for year 1

In the above control plan, the overall budget has not been overspent but there are overspends within some of the individual budget headings. Having checked carefully that no expenditure has been missed or incorrectly entered, you can conclude that the project has £1,880 to transfer to year 2. On an annual basis, the estimated costings for the next year should be checked to take account of price changes. Using a control plan allows management of expenditure under individual budget headings, and the total budget. The Finance department within your organisation may help with the management of the budget and also produce monthly budget statements.

Reviewing the Project

A key activity of project management is to review regularly the status and resources of the project against the project plan. Doing this allows early identification of problems and enables remedial action to be taken. Some funding bodies will require regular progress reports and you may need to keep records of time spent by individuals on the project.

Checklist

1. Do you have an activity and milestone chart (or better still a Gantt chart)?
2. Are you aware of staffing requirements?
3. Do you have a budget and plan for spending?

9) PRESENTING YOUR RESEARCH FINDINGS

- Dissemination
- Publication
- Conference presentation
- Theses

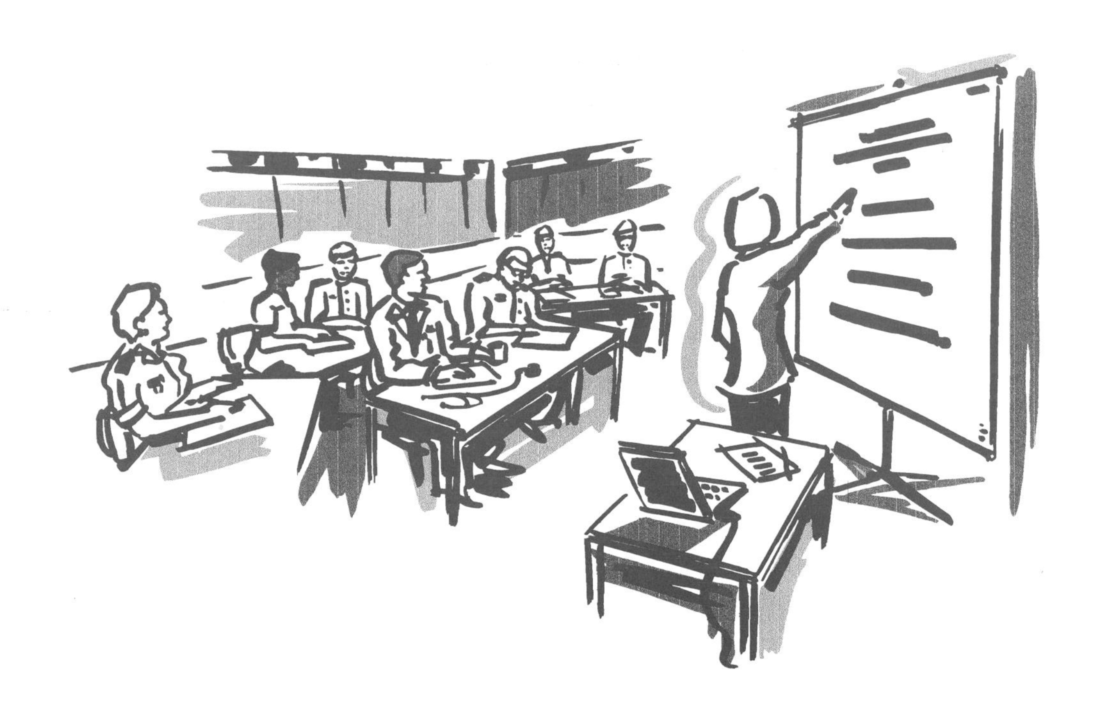

Making the results of your research known to a wide audience is called dissemination. The dissemination of research findings is essential to the research, development and implementation process, including commercial exploitation. The research community has a clear responsibility to justify the use of public funds for research, and dissemination is a major demonstration of this.

All proposed research in the NHS must include a clear intention to publish the results. Without active dissemination, the investment by the NHS and your sponsor will not provide the intended improvements in health care to patients and to the community. Unless research results are disseminated, they will be lost to potential users and other researchers, possibly causing duplication of research effort.

Dissemination is concerned with enhancing the knowledge of decision-makers as they seek to improve the effectiveness of health care practices and policies by basing them upon the best and most up-to-date evidence. Improving knowledge is, however, only one component of changing behaviour, and it is unrealistic to expect that dissemination alone will achieve this. Dissemination is most effective when it is used as part of a wider strategy for changing behaviour. The Cochrane Centre (see Chapter 3) and the York Centre for Reviews and Dissemination, seek to add weight and credibility to research evidence by review and synthesis of multiple research projects.

Dissemination is essentially communication, the essence of which is that the audience understands fully the information or message which is transmitted. It is important therefore to choose an appropriate method of communication for the selected audience, and to ensure that the desired message is concise, succinct and framed in a language and format that the audience can understand.

The target audiences of the dissemination process may include:

- Other researchers within your profession
- Other members of your profession who need to be aware of professional progress
- Other professions and specialities which may be interested in, or affected by, the results
- Managers in Health Authorities and Trusts, and others who are influential in the research, development and implementation process
- Project participants
- Patients
- The public.

It is important to set the findings of the study within the context of accumulated knowledge in the particular field and to indicate clearly the scope and limitations of the work. It may be just as relevant to describe what has not been found out or what was not addressed by the study as to describe the new knowledge generated.

Methods of Dissemination

The main routes for dissemination of research based information are described below.

Publication

The results of a rigorous research study should be published in an appropriate scientific journal. Submissions for publication are examined by a panel of experts in the field (i.e. they are peer-reviewed); acceptable manuscripts are generally returned for corrections and modifications before final approval for inclusion in the journal. Each journal issues guidelines on style, structure and content, and it is important that your manuscript follows these exactly (including the method of identifying references and the appropriate punctuation).

Ideally, a professional study should be published in the profession's own journal. The report of a good quality, properly conducted study will generally enhance the content of a professional journal.

Setting out your findings in an acceptable style and format, combined with the correct use of grammar and punctuation, is essential in order to convey exact and unambiguous meaning. To this end, it is always advisable to consult a suitable textbook, (e.g. Hawkins, 1985; Farquhar & McAllister, 1993) or a guide to writing scientific articles, or to consult an experienced researcher for advice on how to minimise the risk of rejection of a manuscript.

A statistician should be consulted in order that the correct interpretation of statistical analysis can be presented in an appropriate form.

Conferences

Verbal presentations of research work are given at organised conferences, usually after the submission of an abstract in response to a call for papers when the conference is advertised. Presentations may also be given at meetings of professional groups, symposia, lectures, training courses, workshops, or informal meetings which you have arranged yourself.

Whatever the occasion, it is essential to tailor the presentation to suit the audience. Delivering a talk - or 'presenting a paper' - requires skills which usually have to be learned, but problems can be minimised with thorough preparation and rehearsal. Planning the content of the talk and production of the visual or other aids (e.g. videos or slides) may take considerable time, so the process should be started well in advance. Practice your presentation, ideally to colleagues who will understand the subject and who will be constructively critical to improve your performance.

It will pay dividends to read up on the techniques of presentation and how best to design effective 35-millimetre slides and overheads (e.g. Hawkins, 1985).

There are many different types of visual media, e.g. slides, computer presentation packages, overhead projectors and acetates, etc. and therefore it is important to check what facilities are available at your presentation venue before deciding on your choice of media for your presentation.

With regard to **poster displays**, conference organisers always lay down guidelines which must be followed with regard to size and other details. Make sure you are aware of the required materials for fixing the display, and take extra supplies.

Visual appeal is of the essence, so do not expect to include every detail of the study. Try to be available at the display at viewing times to discuss the work and answer questions, and take handouts with contact addresses so that your work can be followed up by interested delegates.

Theses

For academic research, a thesis is the method of presentation of the results of the study. The University's postgraduate department will issue instructions as to the correct format of the document, and the procedure for its submission. These must be followed exactly.

References

Bailey, J. Getting Research into Practice. Proceedings of Getting Research into Practice Workshop. North West R&D Support Network February 1997

Bury, T (ed.). Introduction to Research. London. The Chartered Society of Physiotherapy 1996

Currier, DP. Elements of Research in Physical Therapy (3rd ed.). Baltimore. Williams and Wilkins 1990

Drummond, A. Research Methods for Therapists. London. Chapman and Hall 1996

Farquhar, M & McAllister, G. Publishing Literature Reviews: Why, Who, Where, When and How. Nurse Researcher. Vol. 1. (1), 1993, pp. 64-73

Hawkins, C & Sorgi, M. Research: How to Plan, Speak and Write about It. Berlin. Springer-Verlag 1985

Checklist

1. Have you decided the way(s) in which you are going to disseminate your research findings?
2. Are the methods of dissemination appropriate for your audience?
3. Are there any guidelines available for your method of dissemination, e.g. certain formats/contents for publications or visual aids available for presentations?
4. Have you checked which type of audio visual facilities are available at your presentation venue?

10) USING RESEARCH EVIDENCE

- Evidence-based practice
- Development and implementation
- Critical evaluation and appraisal of research

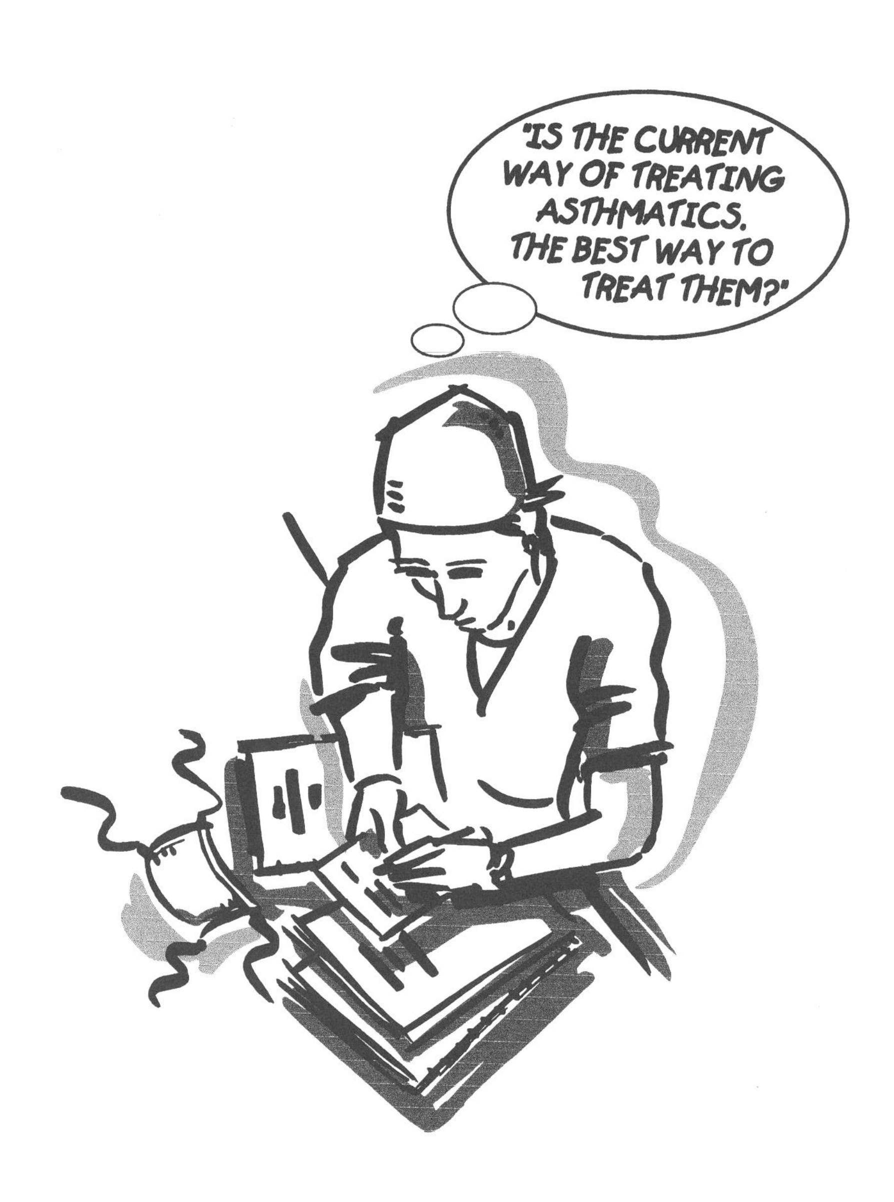

The NHS is actively promoting the use of research findings through its Evidence-Based Medicine initiative (NHS Executive, 1996) and Clinical Governance agenda (NHS Executive, 1998; NHS Executive 1999).

The terms 'evidence-based practice', 'clinical cost-effectiveness' and 'implementing research findings' are all used in relation to improving the quality of health care through the systematic use of research evidence. This is one of the major current issues in the NHS, and a steady stream of research-based evidence is being delivered to fuel these activities.

These activities are complementary to the development end of the research process. Using research evidence is a particular skill which is important not only to researchers but also to all those who are involved in making decisions about health care. Selecting and analysing the best evidence is termed critical appraisal.

Using the results of research to change or influence the way in which health care is delivered is arguably the most important part of the process for the NHS. Without there being a commitment to disseminate and implement the results of a study, the investment by the NHS in the research is wasted.

It follows therefore that, at the beginning of your research, you should be clear about the problem that you intend to address. You should be sure that it is worthwhile and feasible, and that, if the anticipated results are produced, it can be used to change practice for the better. Sometimes, individual pieces of research are able to be developed into a modified or new technique; more often, it is the integration of a number of pieces of research which provides the more powerful argument for change. This is the basis of the 'evidence-based approach' to health care.

Development and the Development Protocol

Doctors, dentists, nurses and managers (the providers of health care and related services) are required to be aware of up-to-date, research-based evidence to support changes in practice; increasingly, Health Authorities are faced with decisions concerning which interventions are effective and should be commissioned, and which are less effective and should not be commissioned.

The value and reliance which can be placed on a piece of research evidence depends upon where it lies within the hierarchy of the different types of evidence. For clinicians and managers, assessment of the quality of outcomes is an essential component of the research, development and implementation process.

Within the NHS, the criteria by which the type and strength of research evidence can be judged have been established by the national R&D Directorate (Bandolier 36, 1997):

- Strong evidence from at least one published systematic review of multiple well-designed randomised controlled trials (RCTs)
- Strong evidence from at least one published properly designed RCT of appropriate size and carried out in an appropriate clinical setting
- Evidence from published well-designed trials without randomisation; or single group pre-post, cohort, time series or matched case-controlled studies
- Evidence from well-designed non-experimental studies from more than one centre or research group
- Opinions of respected authorities, based on clinical evidence; descriptive studies; or reports of expert consensus committees.

It may be assumed therefore that R&D studies which utilise these methodologies are more likely to be accepted for NHS and other funding, and to yield results suitable for development and implementation.

Critical Evaluation and Appraisal of Research

The three steps in the critical appraisal process are described below.

Find

Find the evidence to support the development or implementation of new methods (review the literature), or carry out the research or a pilot study to evaluate new or improved treatment methods (e.g. practice, technology, care process or service provision).

Appraise

Appraise the evidence (using your knowledge of research methods and statistical analysis), answering the following questions:

- Is the study design appropriate?
- Is the sample size suitable?

- Are the instruments valid and reliable? How do you know?
- What are the results?
- Are the data presented correctly?
- Is the statistical analysis appropriate for the data?
- Are the results of the statistical tests presented accurately?
- How valid are the results and are they generalisable?
- Are the results relevant to you and your research question?
- How does the intervention fit the management of the problem?

Act

Initiate a development project.

The process of undertaking a development project is similar in many respects to that of undertaking a research project. The structure and components are similar, and writing a suitable protocol is important for both.

References

Promoting Clinical Effectiveness: A Framework for Action in and through the NHS. NHS Executive 1996

Bandolier 36. 1997, 4, 2 February

A First Class Service, Quality in the new NHS; NHS Executive, 1998

Clinical Governance, Quality in the new NHS; NHS Executive 1999

Useful addresses are:

- **Centre for Evidence-Based Medicine**, University of Oxford, Nuffield Department of Clinical Medicine, The Oxford Radcliffe NHS Trust, Oxford OX3 9DV
- **Bandolier** (newsletter on evidence-based health care), Pain Relief Unit, The Churchill Hospital, Oxford OX3 7LJ - telephone number 01865 226132; Web site: http://www.jr2.ox.ac.uk/Bandolier
- **Effectiveness Matters**, NHS Centre for Reviews and Dissemination, Information Service, University of York, Heslington, York YO1 5DD - telephone number 01904 433707
- **Critical Appraisal Skills Programme (CASP),** Oxford Institute of Health Sciences, PO Box 77, Oxford OX3 7LF
- **DARE** (see NHS Centre for Reviews and Dissemination)

- **Getting Research into Purchasing and Practice (GRiPP),** NHS Executive Anglia and Oxford, Old Road, Headlington, Oxford OX3 7LF - telephone number 01296 310093
- **Promoting Action on Clinical Effectiveness (PACE),** King's Fund Development Centre, 11-13 Cavendish Square, London W1M 0AN - telephone number 0171 307 2400

Checklist

1. Have you the necessary information to appraise the research?
2. Having appraised the research, was it effective?
3. Should a development project be initiated?

Appendix A: Principles Governing the Allocation of Funds from the NHS R&D Levy

(taken from 'R&D Support Funding for NHS Providers')

1. The NHS Executive believes that, in order best to achieve the aims of the NHS R&D Strategy, the following principles should be applied to the allocation of funds from the Levy. They will apply alike to R&D Support Funding for NHS Providers and to the NHS R&D Programme. They will also apply equally to all potential recipients of funds, whatever type and amount of funding they are seeking.

(i) Quality

2. The R&D Levy should only be used to meet the costs of work of good quality, judged by the appropriate prevailing professional standards. It will not, for instance, support work which is unlikely, for whatever reason, to achieve its own objectives.

3. The NHS Executive will therefore seek only to fund R&D activity of good quality. As such, it will expect all recipients of NHS R&D Levy funding to take active steps to ensure their activities achieve appropriate standards. Recipients of funding should be able to demonstrate high levels of quality, and/or systems for improving or (as appropriate) sustaining the quality of their R&D activity. The NHS Executive will also take into account the contribution that potential recipients of funding can make to the general development and spread of R&D expertise and good practice.

4. The NHS R&D Levy should not be used to support unnecessary duplication in R&D effort.

(ii) Ethics

5. The R&D Levy should only be used to support activity which is ethical and has obtained any necessary R&D ethics committee approval.

(iii) Relevance, Impact and Importance

6. The R&D Levy should be used to fund and support activity which is relevant to health gain in the short, medium or long term and which will contribute to the development and implementation within the NHS of evidence-based practice. The views of those working in the NHS must be taken into account in deciding how to use the R&D Levy.

7. The NHS Executive will therefore take steps to ensure the relevance of R&D activity to the NHS' needs (bearing in mind, though not limited to, the NHS' current published Medium Term Priorities and the priorities of local NHS Purchasers and Providers). It will expect potential recipients of funds to do likewise, for example in the selection of subjects for R&D, the methodologies employed and the action taken to disseminate findings.

8. The NHS Executive will also seek evidence that the R&D activity it funds has influenced, or is likely to influence, policy and practice within the NHS in the short, medium or long term. In funding providers of NHS services, the Executive will look for evidence that clinical practice within the provider is appropriately influenced by R&D, and for appropriate links with clinical effectiveness and audit activity.

(iv) Primary Care

9. The NHS Executive believes that R&D activity in primary care is underdeveloped relative to that in other sectors of the NHS. It wishes over time to see this rectified, which will require collaboration with other funders to achieve expansion of existing primary care R&D capacity.

10. The NHS Executive will seek opportunities to use the Levy to promote the development within primary care of good quality R&D activity which is consistent with the other principles set out in this Framework.

(v) Partnership

11. The greatest overall gain from investment in R&D is likely to flow from co-operation between the NHS, universities and others. The R&D Levy should be used in a way which sustains and promotes such co-operation.

12. The NHS Executive will work in partnership with others, and will seek evidence from potential recipients of funds that they too work effectively with appropriate partners, including universities, other NHS and academic bodies, service users, carers, local authorities and industry.

(vi) Support for Non-Commercial Externally Funded R&D

13. The NHS is not alone in funding health and health services R&D. It derives considerable benefit from R&D activity funded by others. The first call on the NHS R&D Levy will therefore be to honour such undertakings as the NHS may make to support non-commercial externally funded R&D.

(vii) Appropriate Disciplinary Mix

14. R&D should draw on and promote the most appropriate mix of skills and expertise, and the R&D Levy should be used to encourage this. The R&D Levy should only be used to support R&D activity undertaken by people or teams with the appropriate skills.

15. The NHS Executive will promote such practice, and will take account of the degree to which potential recipients of funding adopt an appropriately multi-disciplinary approach in selecting, designing and carrying out R&D activity.

(viii) Cost

16. R&D Levy funds should be used as efficiently as possible, so that no more is spent on any activity than is necessary to achieve its objectives.

17. The NHS Executive will seek to use the Levy as efficiently as possible. It will expect all recipients of NHS R&D Levy funds to do likewise, and will favour those best able to do so.

(ix) Integration with other NHS activities

18. R&D is only one of many NHS activities. The use of the R&D Levy should always be integrated with and not disruptive of the operation and development of the NHS as whole.

19. The NHS Executive will therefore take into account in allocating funds the implications for other aspects of NHS services, including patient care, professional training and education. It will seek to balance the needs of each element of NHS activity.

(x) Management

20. Effective management is essential to the achievement of the objectives described in all the above principles. Allocations from the R&D Levy should therefore only be made where they will be well managed, and should favour those recipients able to manage them best. Decisions about what activity to fund should be based on an understanding of its likely long and short-term benefits. Once in progress activity should continue to be appropriately managed.

21. The NHS Executive will seek to manage the Levy well. It will support and encourage the further development of ways of measuring costs, outputs and outcomes to inform decisions about the prioritisation and management of R&D activity. The Executive will in turn expect potential recipients of funds to

demonstrate their own management capacity, not only for funds allocated directly from the Levy, but for all resources and activity which may have a bearing on the effective use of R&D Levy funds. For providers of NHS services, this means that the NHS Executive will be interested not only in the strength of their R&D management, but also its place within their overall management arrangement.

Appendix B: Other Funding Sources

Postal Addresses and Telephone Numbers

Medical Research Council,

20 Park Crescent, London W1N 4AL

Telephone number 0171 636 5422

Economic and Social Research Council,

Polaris House, North Star Avenue, Swindon, Wilts.

Telephone number 01793 413000

The Engineering and Physical Sciences Research Council,

Polaris House, North Star Avenue, Swindon, Wilts.

Telephone number 01793 444347

Biotechnology and Biological Sciences Research Council,

Polaris House, North Star Avenue, Swindon, Wilts.

Telephone number 01793 413256

For European Community funding, the following publication is available from the European Commission in the United Kingdom, 8 Storey's Gate, London SW1 3AT Telephone number 0171 973 1992:
Representation of the European Commission in the UK: Sources of European Community funding. Cardiff. McLays 1995

Web Site Addresses

Association of Medical Research Charities: http://www.mrc.ac.uk/home.html

Research Councils: http://www.nrec.ac.uk/joint_res_councils.html

The Wellcome Trust: http://www.wellcome.ac.uk

There is also a basic funding database (Wisdom) that is part of the Wellcome Trust site. This provides details on funding bodies based on information entered about the type of funding required:

http://www.wellcome.ac.uk/wisdom/schemes.html

Appendix C: The National R&D Priority Areas

These are the programmes identified in March 1998; current information can be obtained from the R&D Department at the Department of Health.

1. Mental Health programme

Mr Tony James, Mental Health Programme Manager, NHS Executive Northern and Yorkshire RO, John Snow House, Durham University Science Park, Durham DH1 3YG.

Telephone number: 0191 301 1332

Fax number: 0191 301 1473

2. Cardiovascular Disease and Stroke programme

Dr Bill Woodbridge, CVD & S Programme Manager, NHS Executive Northern and Yorkshire RO, John Snow House, Durham University Science Park, Durham DH1 3YG.

Telephone number: 0191 224 6108

Fax number: 0191 301 1473

3. Physical and Complex Disabilities programme

Dr Helen Campbell, NHS Executive South and West, Canynge Hall, Whiteladies Road, Bristol BS8 2PR

Telephone number: 0117 928 7258

Fax number: 0117 928 7204

4. Primary and Secondary Care Interface programme

Dr Janet Wisely, NHS Executive North Thames, 40 Eastbourne Terrace, London

W2 3QR

Telephone number: 0171 725 5395

Fax number: 0171 725 5467

5. Heath Technology Assessment programme

Ms Lynn Kerridge, National Co-ordinating Centre for Health, Health Technology Assessment, Boldrewood (Mailpoint 728) University of Southampton, Highfield, Southampton

Telephone number: 01730 595637

Fax number: 01703 595639

6. Cancer programme

Dr Helen Campbell, NHS Executive South and West, Canynge Hall, Whiteladies Road, Bristol BS8 2PR

Telephone number: 0117 928 7258

Fax number: 0117 928 7204

7. Mother and Child Health programme

Dr Janet Wisely, NHS Executive South Thames, 40 Eastbourne Terrace, London W2 3QR

Telephone number: 0171 725 2776

Fax number: 0171 725 2697

8. Methods of implementing research findings

Melanie Baillie-Johnston, National R&D Commissioning Unit (North Thames), R&D Directorate, 40 Eastbourne Terrace, London, W2 3QR

Telephone number: 0171 725 5395

Fax number: 0171 725 5467

9. Asthma programme

Dr Gillian Hastings, National Asthma Campaign, Providence House, Providence Place, London, N1 0NT

Telephone number: 0171 226 2260 X405

Fax number: 0171 704 0704

10. Dental programme

Dr Bill Woodbridge, c/o Ms Marguerite Wood, NHS Executive North West, 930-932 Birchwood Boulevard, Millennium Park, Birchwood, Warrington WA3 7QN

Telephone number: 01925 704133

Fax number: 01925 704266

11. Policy Research programme

Mr R Kirby, Department of Health, R&D Division, Room 403a, Skipton House, Elephant and Castle, London SE1 6LW

Telephone number 0171 972 5631

Glossary of Terms Used in Research

Abstract	A summary of the key features of a project, usually found at the start of journal articles.
Bias	Deviation of the results of a study as a result of flaws in study design. (See 'Sampling bias'.)
Case control studies	Research in which people with a disease/condition and a suitable control are studied. Used usually for studying rare diseases.
CINAHL	Cumulative Index to Nursing and Allied Health Literature, an electronic database which covers research literature published in many nursing and allied health journals.
Cochrane Collaboration	International endeavour which works systematically to find, appraise and review evidence from randomised controlled trials (RCTs). The Collaboration aims to develop and maintain systematic, up-to-date reviews of RCTs of all forms of health care and to make this information available to clinicians and other decision-makers at all levels of health care systems.
Control(s)	The process of holding constant the possible influences on the dependent variable under investigation.
Critical appraisal	The process of assessing and interpreting evidence by systematically considering its validity, results and relevance to your own work.
Data (= plural; singular = datum)	The pieces of information obtained in a research investigation.

Development	The experimental introduction into practice of alternative clinical procedures or methods of care, together with the simultaneous evaluation of their effectiveness, efficiency or both.
Dissemination	Presentation of results to the appropriate target audience, so that others can use your findings. Not restricted to publication in journals.
Ethics	A set of guidelines imposed on a study to ensure that the project will not compromise or upset the subjects in any way.
Experimental design	A method of testing hypotheses which involves manipulating the independent variable(s) in the experimental hypothesis and monitoring what impact this has on the dependent variable. By doing this, cause and effect can be established.
Focus group	A group of interested people guided by a researcher or facilitator in the discussion of a particular topic.
Gantt chart	A tool used in project management. It can be used to help organise the timing of your research activity.
Hypothesis	Supposition that appears to explain a phenomenon and is assumed as a basis of reasoning, experimentation or investigation.
Implementation	The establishment in routine practice of clinical procedures or methods of care for which there is evidence of effectiveness and efficiency. The evidence should be derived from research, development or both. Alternatively, a systematic review could be used as evidence.
Instrument	Device or tool used to take measurements/gather data, e.g. questionnaire.
Intellectual property (IP)	Describes the products of creativity or innovation (such as patents, trademarks or copyright) which do not exist in a physical or tangible form.

Interview	A conversation between a researcher and subject which aims to elicit information relevant to the research area. The interview may be **structured** (follow prescribed topics) or **unstructured** (entirely open).
Literature review	Examination of scientific journals, books, etc. to ascertain the current knowledge or thinking about a topic which may provide the answer to the research question, identify gaps in the knowledge, and give details of methods used.
MEDLINE	An electronic database which summarises research literature published in many medical journals.
Methodology	The type of study design, including the procedures for data collection and analysis.
On-line searching	A search of the worldwide databases to find information relevant to the research topic.
Peer review	The process of assessment of research proposals and items intended for publication, by suitably qualified or experienced reviewers.
Pilot study	Preliminary trial of the research project, with small numbers of subjects, to test for validity and reliability of the instruments (e.g. questionnaires and measuring devices) to be used in the real study.
Placebo	An inactive or dummy treatment given to controls in trials, which appears identical to the active treatment being tested, in order to eliminate psychological effects on the outcome.
Population	The entire set of people with the characteristic under study.
Power calculation	Calculation carried out by a statistician to provide the correct number of subjects required in a study to ensure quality in any statistical analysis carried out.

Protocol	A clearly set out plan of the intended research which includes all relevant details of, and timetable for, the study. This comprehensive plan acts as the basis of information for funding applications, Ethics Committee approval, other permissions, etc.
Qualitative data	Information that is in narrative (non-numerical) form. Can be measured on the nominal scale, i.e. a variable that carries no quantitative information.
Quantitative data	Data collected in the course of a study that is in a quantified (numerical) form. Conveys information about the amount of an attribute, i.e. a variable is measured on the ordinal, interval or ratio scale.
Randomised controlled trial (RCT)	A trial in which subjects are randomly assigned to one of two groups - one (the experimental group) receiving the intervention that is under test, the other (the comparison or control group) receiving an alternative or placebo treatment. The groups are subsequently compared and any differences measured and compared statistically.
Reliability	The extent to which any equipment will give the same result if used on other occasions in similar circumstances.
Research	A systematic approach of inquiry to answer questions or solve problems.
Results	The answers to research questions, obtained through an analysis of the collected data. In a quantitative study, the information obtained through statistical tests.
Sample size	The number of cases (subjects) chosen for a sample from the population to be studied. A statistician should be consulted for a 'power calculation' which will give the number of subjects required.
Sampling	The process of selecting individuals from the population.

Statistical tests	The way in which data are analysed. They show whether results (differences between groups) can be attributed to chance deviations or are real.
Systematic review	A review in which evidence on a topic has been systematically identified, appraised and summarised according to predetermined criteria.
Validity	1) The degree to which an instrument measures what it is intended to measure. 2) Whether the effect on one variable can be attributed to another.
Variable	An attribute of a person or object that varies (i.e. takes on different values).

Bibliography

Title	Topic areas covered
1. Bell, J. Doing Your Research Project: A Guide for First Time Researchers in Education and Social Science. Milton Keynes. Open University Press 1987 Has useful checklists and highlights important points at the end of each chapter. Chapters include questionnaire design and administration as well as interviewing. Chapter 5 focuses on educational research; ideas from this can be transferred to health care research.	B QI
2. Bowling, A. Research Methods in Health: Investigating Health and Health Services. Open University Press 1997 A comprehensive guide to methods used to evaluate health and health care.	G
3. Clamp, C. Resources for Nursing Research: An Annotated Bibliography. London. Library Association Publishing 1993 This is essentially a database of source books for all aspects of the research process directed at nursing. The annotations are brief and coverage is extensive.	L
4. Clifford, C & Gough, S. Nursing Research: A Skills-Based Introduction. Hemel Hempstead. Prentice Hall 1990 This contains a readable section on points to consider when planning a research project. Some of the section on literature-searching is out-of-date, but this chapter does have other useful parts. There is not much pertaining to quantitative research, but it is an adequate introduction to qualitative research. There is a chapter on statistics, providing the basics.	B QI L
5. Cormack, DFS (ed.). The Research Process In Nursing. Oxford. Blackwell Scientific Publications 1991 This book contains a good section on searching for and reviewing literature, as well as an introduction to statistics. Both qualitative and quantitative methodologies are covered.	B L
6. Crombie, IK. The Pocket Guide to Critical Appraisal. London. British Medical Journal Publishing Group 1996 Covers all the necessary topics and has checklists for evaluating articles in general as well as surveys, cohort studies, clinical trials, case-control studies and reviews. There is also a chapter on statistics that is easy to understand.	B

7. Currier, DP. Elements of Research in Physical Therapy (3rd ed.). Baltimore. Williams and Wilkins 1990 This work provides an in-depth introduction to research methods. This American book, written specifically for physical therapists, gives clear guidance in all aspects of the process of undertaking a research study and includes excellent examples to improve the learning process. Suitable for beginners and more experienced researchers in any aspect of health care, it contains many useful references to source documents and is well suited as a text to support academic study and coursework.	B A Qn
8. Cushieri, A & Baker, PR. Introduction to Research in Medical Services. Edinburgh. Churchill Livingstone 1977 A book written for postgraduates in the biomedical or clinical sciences and those about to undertake work in these fields. Although the book is quite old and the data analysis section is rather theoretical and does not reflect the use of computers, it nonetheless would be of interest to its target audience. Has a useful chapter on the presentation of results.	A
9. Dempsey, PA & Dempsey, AD. Nursing Research with Basic Statistical Application. Boston. Jones & Bartlett Publishers 1992 Although aimed at nurses, this book will prove useful to novice researchers of any profession. It covers both qualitative and quantitative research. The chapter on statistics is good but is not suitable for those with no prior statistical knowledge. The section on ethics is more related to United States guidelines, but there is adequate coverage of the general concepts.	S
10. Drummond, A. Research Methods for Therapists. London. Chapman and Hall 1996 A readable book that covers all aspects of research from preparation through to analysis and presentation of data.	G
11. Edwards, A & Talbot, R. The Hard-Pressed Researcher. London. Longman 1994 The book is subtitled 'A Research Handbook for the Caring Professions'. The book's strengths are in the sections on study design, and on the analysis and interpretation of data. However, a straightforward text on statistics would provide similar information. Some statistical tables and a limited glossary are included.	S
12. Goodman, C. Literature Searching and Evidence Interpretation for Assessing Healthcare Practices. Stockholm. The Swedish Council on Health Technology Assessment 1996 A readable guide to selecting research evidence for health technology assessment. It contains a good description of how to set up and carry out a literature search, statistical analysis of the findings and interpretation. It has a good glossary and reading list. It does not include any information on managing and implementing change.	

13. Hawkins, C & Sorgi, M. Research: How to Plan, Speak and Write about It. Berlin. Springer-Verlag 1985 This is an excellent guide to the research process with particular reference to dissemination. It emphasises clarity of expression, and the accuracy of language and data in the presentation of the results and findings of research.	D
14. Hicks, CM. Research for Physiotherapy: Project Design and Analysis. Edinburgh. Churchill Livingstone 1995 Although aimed at physiotherapists, this book can be used by any novice researcher. The chapters on statistics are particularly easy to read and understand.	S G
15. Lumley, JSP. Research: Some Ground Rules. Oxford. Science Publications Good general guide to research, especially useful to those conducting research involving animals (Chapter 6). There is also a chapter on Health and Safety, a topic not always addressed in research methods text books. Has clear and well explained chapters on statistics.	G
16. Moody, LE. Advancing Nursing Sciences through Research. Vols. 1 & 2. Newbury Park. Sage Publications 1990 These two volumes are essentially theory texts which provide advanced discussions of aspects of nursing research. Not for the beginner.	A
17. Polgar, S & Thomas, SA. Introduction to Research in the Health Services. Melbourne. Churchill Livingstone 1988 This book provides a discussion on the scientific method before introducing the relevant parts of the research process. It includes methods of self-assessment of learning such as open questions, true/false questions and multiple choice (with answers).	G
18. Polit, DF. Data Analysis and Statistics for Nursing Research. Stamford. Appleton & Lange 1996 This is a statistics text book which provides the essentials of data analysis and the use of statistics in an easily accessible way. Its range is broad, covering basic terminology and simple descriptive statistics, to computer software printouts and complex multivariate statistics. The book is aimed primarily at nursing research but is equally applicable to any application in health care.	S
19. Reid, N. Health Care Research by Degrees. Oxford. Blackwell Scientific Publications 1993. The researcher is directed through the research process in a logical way. It presents the basis of research in an easily understood form and includes both qualitative and quantitative research. Simple statistical analysis is covered with an introduction to the use of Minitab statistical software.	B Qn Ql

20. Reid, N & Boore, R. Research Methods and Statistics in Health Care. London. Edward Arnold 1987 Norma Reid and Jennifer Bloore's book is aimed primarily at nurses. It provides an introduction to the research process and techniques and deals with the basics of statistical presentation and analysis of data in a clear and easily understood way.	B G
21. Robinson, K, Robinson, H & Hilton, A. Research Awareness. A Programme for Nurses, Midwives and Health Visitors. Module 3: What Is Research? London. HMSO 1992 Uses examples from clinical practice, and activities, which may aid understanding. It is a good introduction to the basic terminology of qualitative and quantitative research.	B Qn Ql
22. Sapsford, R & Abbott, P. Research Methods for Nurses and the Caring Professions. Open University Press 1992 Uses exercise questions throughout the book, although some are not as useful as worked examples. There are helpful chapters pertaining to the use of secondary sources, writing up, putting research into practice, and analysing qualitative data.	B
23. Stewart, M et al. Tools for Primary Care Research. Newbury Park. Sage Publications 1992 This a text book which provides in-depth information on the concepts, techniques, and tools of research. It includes an inventory of psychosocial measurement instruments, many of which have established reliability and validity. This book is aimed at beginners and provides a good basic introduction to research. All the essentials are covered adequately, with good sections on simple statistics and on writing up the results.	B S
24. Usherwood, T. Introduction to Project Management in Health Research: A Guide For New Researchers. Buckingham, Philadelphia. Open University Press 1996 The book introduces and then describes all aspects of managing and undertaking a project. There are also chapters on ethics, obtaining funding and staff recruitment. An example research project is used throughout the book to illustrate the various aspects of project management.	G
25. World Health Organisation. Health Research Methodology: A Guide for Training in Research Methods. Manila. World Health Organisation 1992 This volume is aimed primarily at doctors undertaking clinical trials and epidemiological studies. It contains much useful information about the research process. It is not intended for the new researcher.	Qn

A = Advanced

B = Basic

D = Dissemination

G = General

L = Literature review

Ql = Qualitative research methods

Qn = Quantitative research methods

S = Statistics

Editorial Board

The editorial board also acknowledges the contributions of:

Mr Phil McGinlay (Internet)	Department of Obstetrics and Gynaecology, University of Manchester
Mrs Christina Ireland (Ethics)	Central Manchester Local Research Ethics Committee
Mr Toby Gosden (Health Economics)	National Primary Care R&D Centre